60 HIKES
WITHIN 60 MILES

3rd Edition

WASHINGTON, D.C.

Including Suburban and Outlying Areas of Maryland and Virginia

60 HIKES WITHIN 60 MILES: WASHINGTON, D.C.

Copyright 2017 © Renee Sklarew, Rachel Cooper, Brian Cooper, and Paul Elliott
All rights reserved
Printed in the United States of America
Published by Menasha Ridge Press
Distributed by Publishers Group West
Third edition, first printing

Cataloging-in-Publication Data is available from the Library of Congress.

LCCN 2017006841; ISBN 9781634040822 (pbk.); ISBN 9781634040839 (eISBN)

Cover and text design by Jonathan Norberg
Cover photo: Mason Neck Park © Renee Sklarew
All other photos by Renee Sklarew, Eric Sklarew, Rachel Cooper, and Brian Cooper
Maps by Brian Cooper

MENASHA RIDGE PRESS
An imprint of AdventureKEEN
2204 First Ave. S, Ste. 102
Birmingham, AL 35233

Visit menasharidge.com for a complete listing of our books and for ordering information. Contact us at menasharidge.com, facebook.com/menasharidge, or twitter.com/menasha ridge with questions or comments. To find out more about who we are and what we're doing, visit blog.menasharidge.com.

DISCLAIMER This book is meant only as a guide to select trails in the Washington, D.C., area and does not guarantee hiker safety in any way—you hike at your own risk. Neither Menasha Ridge Press nor the authors of this book are liable for property loss or damage, personal injury, or death that result in any way from accessing or hiking the trails described in the following pages. Please be aware that hikers have been injured in the Washington area. Be especially cautious when walking on or near boulders, steep inclines, and drop-offs, and do not attempt to explore terrain that may be beyond your abilities. To help ensure an uneventful hike, please read carefully the introduction to this book, and perhaps get further safety information and guidance from other sources including the visitor centers or park representatives. Familiarize yourself thoroughly with the areas you intend to visit before venturing out. Ask questions, and prepare for the unforeseen. Familiarize yourself with current weather reports, maps of the area you intend to visit, and any relevant park regulations.

60 HIKES
WITHIN 60 MILES
3rd Edition

WASHINGTON, D.C.

Including Suburban and Outlying Areas of Maryland and Virginia

Renee Sklarew and Rachel Cooper
Prior edition by Paul Elliott

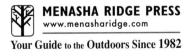

MENASHA RIDGE PRESS
www.menasharidge.com
Your Guide to the Outdoors Since 1982

60 Hikes Within 60 Miles: Washington, D.C.

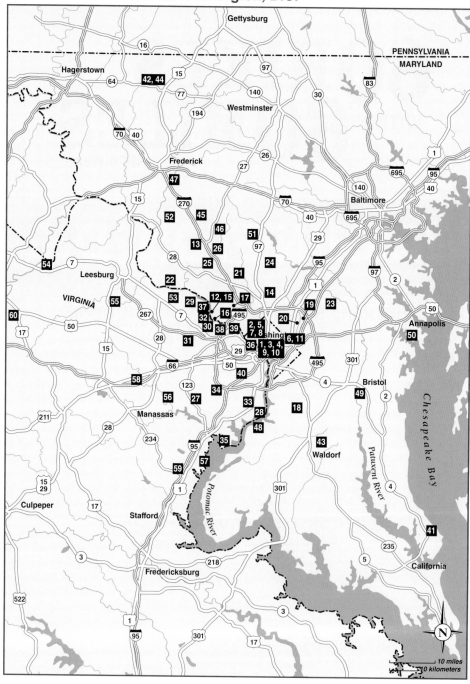

TABLE OF CONTENTS

CLOSE-IN VIRGINIA SUBURBS
(Alexandria, Arlington, and Fairfax Counties) 130

RURAL MARYLAND (Parts of Montgomery and Prince George's
Counties; Anne Arundel, Calvert, and Frederick Counties) 190

ACKNOWLEGMENTS

We are grateful to Paul Elliott for creating the first two editions of this book. We understand that it is much beloved by many Washington, D.C.–area hiking enthusiasts. Like Paul, we appreciate the assistance we received at the various parks and the expertise of many local guides and rangers.

While we included many of Paul's recommended hikes from previous editions, we decided to start almost completely fresh. We chose our own trails, made our own maps, and dropped and added parks for various reasons. In making our choices, we focused on appealing to a wide range of hikers, with options that range from easy to challenging, all of which can be accomplished on a day trip.

The most significant difference you will find are the new maps. Brian Cooper has profiled the trails we recorded with our Garmin eTrex units, which record elevations, distance, waypoints, and trailheads. Using the Garmin BaseCamp software application, Brian made sure every hike corresponds accurately with the narrative directions provided.

Before heading out on the trails, we relied on maps provided by the national, state, and local park services. We made sure to research where we were going and download any maps available to help us venture forth. Even with our park maps, there will be occasions when you will, like us, get a little lost or feel unsure about the turns you make. Out in the wild, some trails are not well marked and can be difficult to follow, but that is part of the adventure.

We hail the millions of volunteers who help maintain the parks, either with financial contributions or physical improvements, such as marking blazes, building structures that support the trail, and keeping the paths clear. Additional salutes go to the landscape shapers and environmental stewards, historians and visionaries, bloggers and hiking clubs that help introduce so many people to our treasured natural landscapes. They all have our collective thanks.

For the third edition, with its many new hikes and revised old ones, we wish to thank our intrepid family and friends who have been out on the trails with us, waiting patiently for us to document the waypoints, record directions, pose in pictures, and give us the moral support to finish this book. Special thanks go to Renee's husband, Eric, who taught her about the native plants of this region. Thanks also to Scott McGrew for his work translating our GPS data into user-friendly maps. We also appreciate Tim Jackson for his trust in our ability to take on this challenging assignment; Kate Johnson for her sharp eyes, diligent editing skills and patient guidance; and to Menasha Ridge Press editor Holly Cross, who put all the pieces together to make it print-ready.

—Renee Sklarew, Rachel Cooper, and Brian Cooper

FOREWORD

Welcome to Menasha Ridge Press's 60 Hikes Within 60 Miles, a series designed to provide hikers with information needed to find and hike the very best trails and other hiking routes in and around cities usually underserved by good guidebooks.

Our strategy is simple: First, find hikers who know the area and love to hike. And second, ask these people to spend a year hiking, mapping, photographing, and describing the very best hiking routes around in terms of difficulty, scenery, condition, elevation change, and all other categories of information that are important to hikers. "On each hike, pretend you are a new hiker to the area and think about what any hiker would want to know," we tell each author. "Imagine their questions; be clear in your answers."

Paul Elliott set the groundwork with first edition of this book. This is the third edition, the work of two hikers and a technology whiz who sought out hikes for all types of hikers. From urban hikes that make use of parklands and streets to flora- and fauna-rich treks along the Potomac River to aerobic outings in the mountains, this edition provides hikers (and walkers) with a great variety of hikes—all within roughly 60 miles of D.C.

You'll get more out of this book if you take a moment to read the Introduction (page 1), which explains how to read the hike profiles and listings. The 60 Hikes by Category chart (page xiv) will help you choose an appropriate destination based on your specific interests and needs. The flora and fauna section provides an overview of the region's native wildlife and vegetation. And though this is a where-to, not a how-to, guide, those of you who have not hiked extensively will find the Introduction of particular value.

As much for the opportunity to free the mind as to free the body, let us direct you to hikes that elevate you above the urban commotion.

All the best,

The Editors at Menasha Ridge Press

The maps in this book have been produced with care using the latest GPS receivers and Geographic Information System (GIS) software. When used with the hike descriptions, they will successfully direct you to the trailhead and keep you on course during the hike. However, because trail maintenance, new construction, storm or flood damage, and other factors can cause trails to change, we recommend consulting the online and/or physical resources referenced herein before venturing forth.

Although recreational GPS technology has improved dramatically over the past five years, coordinates are still accurate only to about 100 feet per measurement. Accuracy can be further impaired by poor satellite reception due to heavy foliage, canyons (both urban and natural), and upper atmospheric disturbances. Therefore, cumulative trail distance measurements may vary by 10% or more. This is a long-winded way of saying that your GPS mileage may vary. If you are using a fitness tracker or pedometer to measure your hiking distance, then your distances may vary from ours.

Our hiking times are based on our own hikes and include time for taking pictures, enjoying the vistas, or eating lunch. Although we typically hiked at a speed of 3–5 miles per hour when actually walking, our cumulative average speeds were closer to 1.5–2 miles per hour. As with our distances, your hiking times may vary. Always check the weather before your start out, dress appropriately, and carry enough water to keep yourself adequately hydrated.

In addition to a map and trail guide, it's a good idea to take along a compass and/or GPS unit (and know how to use all of them).

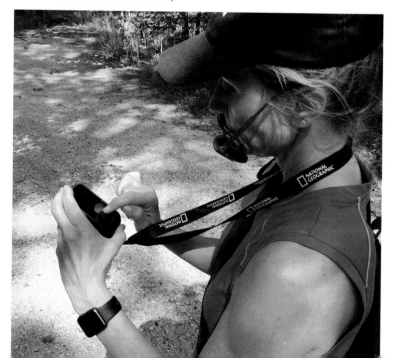

Directional arrows

Featured trail

Alternate trail

Freeway

Highway with bridge

Minor road

Boardwalk

Stairs

Unpaved road

Park/forest

Body of water

River/creek/
intermittent stream

✈ Airport

⚓ Amphitheater

🕺 Baseball field

🏖 Beach access

🗋 Bench

🚤 Boat launch

⛰ Campground

🛶 Canoe access

✝ Cemetery

🔧 Dam

🥛 Drinking water

🔥 Fire pit

🎣 Fishing access

✂ Footbridge

❋ Garden

•—• Gate

● General point of interest

🏌 Golf course

⛸ Ice-skating rink

? Information kiosk

⚓ Marina

Marsh

Ⓜ Metro station

🗼 Monument

Observation tower

► One-way (road)

△ Overlook

⌂ Park office

🅿 Parking

▲ Peak/hill

🏕 Picnic area

🏕 Picnic shelter

🚽 Pit toilets

🛝 Playground

△ Primitive campsite

🚻 Restrooms

🏠 Scenic view

⌐ Shelter

⚽ Soccer field

🐴 Stable

🎾 Tennis court

🚶 Trailhead

🏚 Viewing platform

// Waterfall/cascades

♿ Wheelchair-accessible

PREFACE

"I like walking because it is slow, and I suspect that the mind, like the feet, works at about three miles an hour. If this is so, then modern life is moving faster than the speed of thought, or thoughtfulness."

—Rebecca Solnit,
Wanderlust: A History of Walking, page 10

In researching and writing this edition of the book, we had two basic objectives in mind. One was to tell or remind both local residents and visitors about the exceptional hiking opportunities available in the Washington, D.C., metropolitan area—and not just in exurbia and suburbia but also in the city itself. The metro area has something to offer just about anyone with an interest in hiking. Taken together, these trails reflect the area's rich diversity of landscape, parklands, wildlife, city life, historical heritage, cultural resources, and recreational opportunity, as well as its tradition of preservation and conservation. What's more, hiking in the metro area is very much a rewarding four-season enterprise.

Our other objective was to provide residents and visitors with a reliable means of exploring the local world of hiking on their own—without relying on organized

As you explore Washington, D.C., wetland environments, you're likely to see plenty of geese enjoying them, too.

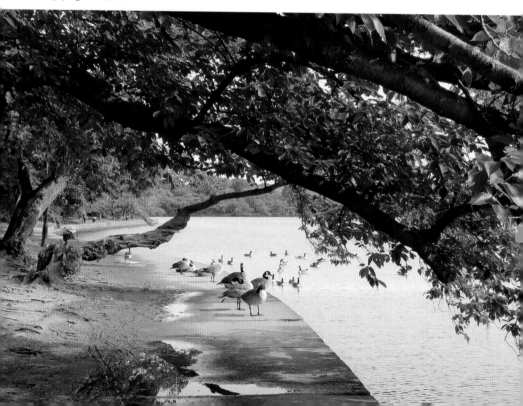

group outings. Our intent was to present them with tempting choices, tell them what to expect, motivate them to get out there, and enable them to experience on-course, safe, and enjoyable outings. We urge readers to select their hikes wisely; read the words and maps attentively; and take along a cell phone, compass, and maybe a companion. We also warn hikers that trail signage and landmarks sometimes disappear and guidebooks tend to get out of date.

For Paul Elliott's first edition, he created an eclectic mix of 60 hikes that ranged in location from the central city to and through the suburbs, incorporating the foothills and mountains in the west and the lowlands and wetlands in the east. The hikes fell into two categories: traditional hikes in already-popular hiking locales and hidden gem–style hikes in underused areas. For this edition, we scouted out Paul's recommendations and eliminated some that catered to cyclists rather than hikers. We sought out places that showcased the best of the region's wild spaces. Last, we wanted our hikes to be in the form of day trips, not backpacking expeditions. We hiked together for some, but mostly split the trails to complete the book in a timely fashion. Hiking on our own, often on weekdays when the parks were not heavily trafficked, offered peace and quiet. The downside was the lack of people to ask for directions. This required us to research the trails ahead of time and rely on maps to find our way.

Here's what it takes to write such a book: time, a reliable car, a cell phone, a GPS unit, good descriptive skills, strong legs, excellent hiking boots, a lightweight camera, and persistence. Because of this experience, we are more determined than ever to preserve and protect our public spaces and promote the acquisition of more. We deeply appreciate the vital role played by our federal, state, and local agencies and especially by local nonprofits such as the Potomac Appalachian Trail Club (the area's chief trail builder and maintainer), the Appalachian Trail Conservancy, the Potomac Conservancy, the C&O Canal Association, and the Potomac Heritage Trail Association, plus the other organizations listed in Appendix A.

If you have any comments or suggestions for future editions, please write to us on our Facebook page: facebook.com/60HikesWithin60MilesDC

—Renee Sklarew and Rachel Cooper, authors,
with Brian Cooper, map specialist

60 HIKES BY CATEGORY

REGION Hike Number/Hike Name	page	Within the Beltway	Minor Elevation Gain	Major Elevation Gain	Flora or Fauna	Bodies of Water	Overlooks with Views	Historic Sites
WASHINGTON, D.C.								
1 Anacostia Riverwalk Trail	16	✓	✓			✓		✓
2 Capital Crescent Trail: Fletcher's Cove to Georgetown Waterfront Park	20	✓	✓			✓		✓
3 Columbia Island	24	✓	✓			✓		✓
4 East Potomac Park and Jefferson Memorial	29	✓	✓			✓		✓
5 Glover Archbold Park Trail and Potomac Heritage Trail	33	✓	✓		✓	✓		✓
6 Kenilworth Aquatic Gardens and the Anacostia Riverwalk Trail	37	✓	✓		✓	✓		✓
7 Rock Creek Park: Boulder Bridge Trail	42	✓		✓	✓	✓	✓	✓
8 Rock Creek Park: Northern Section	47	✓	✓					✓
9 Theodore Roosevelt Island National Memorial	52	✓	✓		✓	✓	✓	✓
10 Tidal Basin and West Potomac Park	57	✓	✓			✓		✓
11 United States National Arboretum	62	✓	✓		✓			✓
CLOSE-IN MARYLAND SUBURBS								
12 Billy Goat Trail: Sections A and B	68	✓		✓	✓	✓	✓	
13 Black Hill Regional Park	72			✓	✓	✓		✓
14 Brookside Gardens and Wheaton Regional Park	76		✓		✓	✓		✓
15 C&O Canal Towpath: Great Falls to Angler's Inn with Olmsted Island	80	✓	✓		✓	✓	✓	✓
16 C&O Canal Towpath: Old Angler's Inn to Carderock Recreation Area	85		✓		✓	✓	✓	✓
17 Cabin John Regional Park	89	✓	✓		✓	✓		
18 Cosca Regional Park	93		✓		✓			
19 Greenbelt Park	97		✓		✓	✓		
20 Lake Artemesia Natural Area and Northeast Branch Trail	101		✓		✓	✓		
21 Lake Needwood and Maryland's Rock Creek Regional Park	105		✓		✓	✓		
22 McKee-Beshers Wildlife Management Area	109		✓		✓			✓
23 Patuxent Research Refuge: Cash Lake Trail	113		✓		✓	✓		
24 Sandy Spring Underground Railroad Trail: Woodlawn Manor Cultural Park	117		✓		✓			✓
25 Seneca Creek State Park: Lake Shore Trail	122			✓		✓		✓
26 Seneca Greenway Trail: Frederick Road (MD 355) to Brink Road	126		✓		✓			✓

REGION Hike Number/Hike Name	page	Within the Beltway	Minor Elevation Gain	Major Elevation Gain	Flora or Fauna	Bodies of Water	Overlooks with Views	Historic Sites
CLOSE-IN VIRGINIA SUBURBS								
27 Burke Lake Park Trail	132		✓			✓		
28 Difficult Run Stream Valley Park: Gerald Connolly Cross County Trail	135			✓	✓	✓	✓	
29 Fort Hunt Park and Mount Vernon Trail	139		✓			✓		✓
30 Fraser Preserve	143		✓		✓	✓		
31 Glade Stream Valley Park	147		✓			✓		
32 Great Falls Park	151		✓		✓	✓	✓	✓
33 Huntley Meadows Park	157		✓		✓	✓	✓	
34 Lake Accotink Park Trail	161		✓			✓		
35 Mason Neck State Park and National Wildlife Refuge	165		✓		✓	✓	✓	
36 Potomac Overlook Regional Park and Nature Center	170	✓	✓		✓	✓	✓	
37 Riverbend Park and the Potomac Heritage Trail	174			✓	✓	✓	✓	✓
38 Scott's Run Nature Preserve	178		✓		✓	✓	✓	
39 Turkey Run Park and the Potomac Heritage Trail	182	✓		✓	✓	✓	✓	✓
40 Winkler Botanical Preserve	186	✓	✓		✓	✓		
RURAL MARYLAND								
41 Calvert Cliffs State Park	192		✓		✓	✓	✓	
42 Catoctin Mountain Park	197			✓	✓		✓	✓
43 Cedarville State Forest	201		✓		✓	✓		
44 Cunningham Falls State Park	204		✓		✓	✓	✓	
45 Jug Bay Wetlands Sanctuary	208		✓		✓	✓	✓	
46 Little Bennett Regional Park	213		✓		✓	✓		
47 Magruder Branch Trail and Lower Magruder Trail	217		✓			✓		
48 Monocacy National Battlefield	220		✓			✓	✓	✓
49 National Colonial Farm at Piscataway Park	225		✓		✓	✓	✓	✓
50 Quiet Waters Park	230		✓			✓	✓	
51 Rachel Carson Conservation Park	233		✓		✓	✓		
52 Sugarloaf Mountain	237			✓	✓		✓	✓

REGION Hike Number/Hike Name	page	Within the Beltway	Minor Elevation Gain	Major Elevation Gain	Flora or Fauna	Bodies of Water	Overlooks with Views	Historic Sites
RURAL VIRGINIA								
53 Algonkian Regional Park	244	✓			✓	✓	✓	
54 Appalachian Trail: Raven Rocks	248		✓	✓		✓		
55 Banshee Reeks Nature Preserve	252	✓			✓	✓	✓	✓
56 Bull Run–Occoquan Trail	256	✓			✓	✓		
57 Leesylvania State Park	260	✓			✓	✓	✓	
58 Manassas National Battlefield Park	265	✓			✓	✓	✓	✓
59 Prince William Forest Park	270	✓			✓			
60 Sky Meadows State Park	274			✓	✓	✓	✓	✓

More Hikes by Category

REGION Hike Number/Hike Name	Bikeable	Wheelchair Traversable	MetroRail or MetroBus	1 to 5 Miles	5 to 10 Miles	Longer Options	National Park	Kid Friendly
WASHINGTON, D.C.								
1 Anacostia Riverwalk Trail	✓	✓	✓	✓		✓		✓
2 Capital Crescent Trail: Fletcher's Cove to Georgetown Waterfront Park	✓		✓		✓	shorter options		
3 Columbia Island	partial		✓	✓				
4 East Potomac Park and Jefferson Memorial	✓		✓		✓	✓	✓	✓
5 Glover Archbold Park Trail and Potomac Heritage Trail			✓	✓		✓	✓	✓
6 Kenilworth Aquatic Gardens and the Anacostia Riverwalk Trail		partial	✓	✓		shorter options	✓	✓
7 Rock Creek Park: Boulder Bridge Trail			✓	✓		✓	✓	
8 Rock Creek Park: Northern Section			✓		✓	✓	✓	
9 Theodore Roosevelt Island National Memorial	partial	partial	✓	✓		shorter options	✓	✓
10 Tidal Basin and West Potomac Park			✓	✓		✓	✓	✓
11 United States National Arboretum	✓	✓			✓	shorter options	✓	✓

REGION Hike Number/Hike Name	Bikeable	Wheelchair Traversable	MetroRail or MetroBus	1 to 5 Miles	5 to 10 Miles	Longer Options	National Park	Kid Friendly
CLOSE-IN MARYLAND SUBURBS								
12 Billy Goat Trail: Sections A and B				✓		✓	✓	
13 Black Hill Regional Park	✓	✓			✓	shorter options		✓
14 Brookside Gardens and Wheaton Regional Park		partial		✓		shorter options		✓
15 C&O Canal Towpath: Great Falls to Angler's Inn with Olmsted Island	✓	✓		✓		✓	✓	✓
16 C&O Canal Towpath: Old Angler's Inn to Carderock Recreation Area	✓			✓		✓	✓	✓
17 Cabin John Regional Park				✓		✓		✓
18 Cosca Regional Park		partial		✓				✓
19 Greenbelt Park			✓	✓		✓	✓	
20 Lake Artemesia Natural Area and Northeast Branch Trail	✓	✓	✓	✓		✓		✓
21 Lake Needwood and Maryland's Rock Creek Regional Park	partial			✓				✓
22 McKee-Beshers Wildlife Management Area	✓				✓	✓		
23 Patuxent Research Refuge: Cash Lake Trail		partial		✓		✓		✓
24 Sandy Spring Underground Railroad Trail: Woodlawn Manor Cultural Park				✓		shorter options		✓
25 Seneca Creek State Park: Lake Shore Trail				✓				✓
26 Seneca Greenway Trail: Frederick Road (MD 355) to Brink Road	✓				✓	✓		
CLOSE-IN VIRGINIA SUBURBS								
27 Burke Lake Park Trail	✓	partial			✓			✓
28 Difficult Run Stream Valley Park: Gerald Connolly Cross County Trail				✓		✓	✓	✓
29 Fort Hunt Park and Mount Vernon Trail	✓	partial			✓			
30 Fraser Preserve			✓	✓		shorter options		✓
31 Glade Stream Valley Park	✓			✓		shorter options		✓
32 Great Falls Park		partial		✓		✓	✓	✓
33 Huntley Meadows Park		partial		✓				✓
34 Lake Accotink Park Trail	✓			✓		✓		✓
35 Mason Neck State Park and National Wildlife Refuge		partial		✓				✓
36 Potomac Overlook Regional Park and Nature Center		partial	✓	✓		✓		✓

REGION Hike Number/Hike Name	Bikeable	Wheelchair Traversable	MetroRail or MetroBus	1 to 5 Miles	5 to 10 Miles	Longer Options	National Park	Kid Friendly
CLOSE-IN VIRGINIA SUBURBS *(continued)*								
37 Riverbend Park and the Potomac Heritage Trail				✓		✓	✓	✓
38 Scott's Run Nature Preserve				✓		✓		✓
39 Turkey Run Park and the Potomac Heritage Trail			✓	✓		✓	✓	✓
40 Winkler Botanical Preserve				✓		✓		✓
RURAL MARYLAND								
41 Calvert Cliffs State Park				✓		✓		✓
42 Catoctin Mountain Park					✓	✓	✓	
43 Cedarville State Forest	✓				✓	shorter options		✓
44 Cunningham Falls State Park				✓		✓		✓
45 Jug Bay Wetlands Sanctuary				✓		✓		
46 Little Bennett Regional Park					✓	✓		
47 Magruder Branch Trail and Lower Magruder Trail	✓			✓		✓		
48 Monocacy National Battlefield		✓		✓		shorter options	✓	✓
49 National Colonial Farm at Piscataway Park				✓			✓	
50 Quiet Waters Park	✓	✓		✓				✓
51 Rachel Carson Conservation Park				✓		✓		
52 Sugarloaf Mountain				✓		✓		✓
RURAL VIRGINIA								
53 Algonkian Regional Park		partial		✓		✓		✓
54 Appalachian Trail: Raven Rocks					✓	✓		
55 Banshee Reeks Nature Preserve	✓			✓		✓		
56 Bull Run–Occoquan Trail	✓			✓		✓		
57 Leesylvania State Park	partial	partial		✓		✓		✓
58 Manassas National Battlefield Park					✓	shorter options	✓	
59 Prince William Forest Park					✓		✓	✓
60 Sky Meadows State Park				✓		✓		✓

INTRODUCTION

Welcome to *60 Hikes Within 60 Miles: Washington, D.C.* If you're new to hiking or even if you're a seasoned trailsmith, take a few minutes to read the following introduction. We explain how this book is organized and how to use it.

What's in Each Hike Listing

Each hike contains a brief overview of the trail, a description of the route from start to finish, key at-a-glance information—from the trail's distance and configuration to contacts for local information—GPS trailhead coordinates, directions for driving to the trailhead area, and a note about nearby and related activities. Each profile also includes a trail map and elevation profile (if the elevation gain is 100 feet or more).

IN BRIEF

This synopsis offers a snapshot of what to expect along the way, mostly in general terms of the hike's location and its chief attractions for hikers.

KEY AT-A-GLANCE INFORMATION

This box gives you a quick idea of the hike's specifics with 17 or 18 basic elements.

LENGTH Specifies the hike's length from start to finish. For many hikes, the authors note that there are shorter and longer options. The options are explained in the hike description, and you can use them to customize the hike to match your ability, inclination, or time constraints.

CONFIGURATION Characterizes the hiking route's overall shape if it could be seen from overhead. Most of the hikes are loops, out-and-backs, or modifications of these two types.

DIFFICULTY Indicates the degree of effort an average hiker will likely need to make. Using a simple formula of distance and elevation change, the hikes range from "Very Easy" to "Difficult," as explained in the Preface.

SCENERY Summarizes what you can expect in general terms of terrain, vegetation, land use, water bodies, and views.

EXPOSURE Reveals how much sunshine will land on your shoulders on a clear day. The exposure scale uses "open" and "shady" proportionately and makes allowance for the effects of trees, cliffs, buildings, and seasons.

TRAFFIC Indicates how busy the trail might be on an average day. Trail traffic, of course, will vary from day to day and season to season.

TRAIL SURFACE Most trail surfaces are paved, dirt, grass, or rock. The trail design and materials influence the difficulty of a hike. Note that paved trails are the easiest, especially in wet weather conditions.

HIKING TIME Provides a practical range based on the authors' own experiences and perceptions of the average hiker.

DRIVING DISTANCE Indicates driving distance from Washington, D.C., using the U. S. Capitol as a starting point.

SEASON Names the best times of year for doing the hike, in the authors' opinions.

ACCESS Reveals the days and times of day when the route is officially open, and whether hikers must pay usage fees or obtain permission to hike.

WHEELCHAIR TRAVERSABLE Notes whether the trail is wheelchair compatible. In some cases, wheelchairs will need to have larger wheels that can move over unpaved but hard-packed surfaces.

MAPS Identifies maps that usefully supplement the trail map in each hike listing, and identifies some map sources. Websites beginning with "tinyurl.com" are aliases we created to shorten long URLs. Entering this shortened version will redirect you to the map's website.

FACILITIES Lists toilets, public phones, and water sources available along or near the hiking route or simply specifies "None."

CONTACT Provides phone numbers and websites, where applicable, for up-to-date information on trail conditions.

LOCATION Identifies the city and state in which the trail is located.

COMMENTS Reminds you about park or gate closings, the possibility of flooding or freezing, hunting seasons, and other factors that could affect your plans.

DIRECTIONS Leads you to the trailhead. Follow these driving directions carefully, with the locator map in hand, to get to the trailhead and park legally. Some hikes include public-transportation options.

DESCRIPTION

This is the heart of each hike listing. Here, the authors present what is essentially a combination of essay and hiking guide, in which they create a vivid and concise picture of the venue's natural and human history and provide easy-to-follow instructions and a map to keep you on course. Ultimately, the description is your chief tool in deciding what hikes to try—and which ones to repeat.

NEARBY/RELATED ACTIVITIES

Each hike listing includes suggestions for other things to do, including other hikes listed in the book. The suggestions might include places to detour privately, swim, picnic, bird-watch, row, take a ranger-led tour or sunset boat ride, dine indoors, pick fruit, attend an outdoor play or concert, sample a festival, dig into history, explore an oddball museum, hike by moonlight, stargaze, ride a horse (on a trail or antique carousel), find an ice-cream shop, or meditate in a peaceful park.

ELEVATION PROFILES

For trails with significant changes in elevation, the hike description will contain a detailed elevation profile that corresponds directly to the trail map. This graphical element provides a quick look at the trail from the side, enabling you to visualize how the trail rises and falls. Varying height scales provide an accurate image of each hike's climbing challenge. Elevation profiles for loop hikes show the total route; those for out-and-back hikes show only one way.

GPS COORDINATES

In addition to highly specific trail outlines, this book also includes the latitude (north) and longitude (west) coordinates for each trailhead. The latitude–longitude grid system is likely quite familiar to you, but here's a refresher.

Imaginary lines of latitude—called parallels and approximately 69 miles apart from each other—run horizontally around the globe. Each parallel is indicated by degrees from the equator (established to be 0°): up to 90°N at the North Pole and down to 90°S at the South Pole.

Imaginary lines of longitude—called meridians—run perpendicular to lines of latitude and are likewise indicated by degrees. Starting from 0° at the Prime Meridian in Greenwich, England, they continue to the east and west until they meet 180° later at the International Date Line in the Pacific Ocean. At the equator, longitude lines are also approximately 69 miles apart, but that distance narrows as the meridians converge toward the North and South Poles.

In this book, latitude and longitude are expressed in degree–decimal minute format. For example, the coordinates for Hike 1 (page 16) are as follows: N38° 53.343' W77° 01.690'. For more on GPS technology, visit usgs.gov.

Weather

The Washington, D.C., metropolitan area has a generally temperate climate that favors year-round hiking, though deep freezes and major storms sometimes occur in the winter, and the often hot and humid summers take some getting used to. It's also common for thunderstorms to begin after a hot summer day, so keep an eye on the sky. Get off the trail as soon as possible if you see threatening clouds or hear thunder.

If you make prudent decisions about which of these 60 hikes to try, what to take with you, and what the weather is likely to be, you can count on being able to hike enjoyably and safely on most days of the year.

During the winter, early-morning temperatures are usually near the freezing mark, and frosts are not uncommon throughout much of the area. Remember that winter weather in the mountains tends to be more severe than elsewhere, so pay attention to mountain-weather forecasts. Some winters bring little or no snow— and some bring warm spells. Even a mild winter tends to be a gray season of short days, but winter hiking in the area has its devotees, who enjoy the absence of leaves, insects, and crowds and who delight in the opened-up vistas.

AVERAGE DAILY TEMPERATURES BY MONTH IN WASHINGTON, D.C.						
MONTH	JAN	FEB	MAR	APR	MAY	JUN
High	42° F	44° F	53° F	64° F	75° F	83° F
Low	27° F	28° F	35° F	44° F	54° F	63° F
MONTH	JUL	AUG	SEP	OCT	NOV	DEC
High	87° F	84° F	78° F	67° F	55° F	45° F
Low	68° F	66° F	59° F	48° F	38° F	29° F

Source: usclimatedata.com/climate/district-of-columbia/united-states/3178

On the hottest days of summer, from late July to early September, try to go hiking first thing in the morning, and look for hikes that have heavy shade or that are in the mountains, where temperatures are routinely lower (generally, one degree lower for every 1,000 feet of elevation gain). Keep in mind that even late in the day, the temperature and humidity won't have dropped enough to be really comfortable. As mentioned earlier, be wary of thunderstorms, which are the area's most common weather hazard in summer.

All in all, the best hiking weather in the Washington area occurs in the fall and spring. Autumn can be glorious, especially from September to early December, during Indian summer. With the return of spring, between about mid-March and mid-May, comes balmy weather, the reawakening of the plant world, and the reappearance of songbirds and lots of hikers.

Learn About Using Maps

The maps in this book have been produced with great care and, when used with the hike descriptions, will direct you to the trailhead and keep you on course during the hike. However, for superior detail and other valuable information about the terrain you'll be traversing, you should also use digital and topographical maps to confirm that the details are up-to-date and get specific directions from your location.

If you're new to hiking, you might be wondering, "What's a topographic map?" In short, a topo map indicates not only linear distance but also elevation, using contour lines. Contour lines spread across the map like dozens of intricate spiderwebs. Each line represents a particular elevation, and at the base of each map, a contour's interval designation is given. If the contour interval is 200 feet, then the height difference between each contour line is 200 feet. Follow five contour lines up on the same map, and the elevation has increased by 1,000 feet.

You can find topo maps at local outdoors stores and some bike shops, as well as online at many websites. For the 7.5-minute USGS maps, visit the USGS website topomaps.usgs.gov. These and other topo maps—and aerial photographs—can also be found at topozone.com. Another valuable map resource in Washington is the Library of Congress, which has a treasure trove of maps that the public can use and photocopy.

Practice Trail Etiquette

Whether you're on a city walk or a long hike, remember that great care and resources (from nature as well as from tax dollars) have gone into creating the trails and paths. Maintaining them begins with you, the hiker. Treat the trail, wildlife, flora, and your fellow hikers with respect. Here are a few general ideas to keep in mind while hiking:

➤ **Hike on open trails only.** Respect trail and road closures (ask if you're not sure), avoid trespassing on private land, and obtain any required permits or authorization. Leave gates as you found them or as marked.

➤ **Leave no trace of your visit other than footprints.** Be sensitive to the land beneath your feet. This also means staying on the existing trails and not creating any new ones. Be sure to pack out what you pack in. No one likes to see trash someone else has left behind. Also, consider packing out at least some of the trash you find along the trail (in the D.C. area, many parks no longer provide trash receptacles).

➤ **Never spook animals.** Give animals extra room and time to adjust to you.

➤ **Plan ahead. Know your equipment, your ability, and the area in which you are hiking, and prepare accordingly.** Be self-sufficient at all times; carry necessary supplies for changes in weather or other conditions. A well-executed trip is a satisfaction to you and not a burden or offense to others.

➤ Be respectful of and courteous to everyone you meet while hiking.

Be Sure You Have and Drink Enough Water

One of the keys to hiking both enjoyably and safely in the Washington area is keeping well hydrated. So be sure to take along enough water. How much is enough? The answer depends chiefly on the length and duration of the hike and the ambient temperature. One year-round standard recommended by some local hiking clubs is to carry at least 1 quart for every 5 miles to be covered. During the summer, your thirst will increase substantially.

Try to start any hike with potable water. Some hikes in this book have drinking water available at the trailhead or along the way. But if you must use water that's not from a reliable tap, make sure you purify it; otherwise, you run the risk of infection. That's because waterways throughout the area—including high-mountain streams and springs—can be sources of unwelcome bacteria (such as giardia, cryptosporidium, and *E. coli*), as well as viruses and other pollutants.

All in all, the best way to stay safe is to bring water from home with you. The pleasures of hiking—and the displeasure of getting sick—make such relatively minor efforts worth every one of the minutes involved.

Useful Things to Take on the Hike

Choose sensibly from the following list:

- ➤ Bandanna
- ➤ Companion or companions
- ➤ Cell phone
- ➤ Cold-weather clothing (*such as hat, gloves, extra layers, dry socks*)
- ➤ Compass
- ➤ First aid options such as bandages for blisters
- ➤ Flashlight (plus extra batteries)
- ➤ Food, such as an energy bar or protein snack
- ➤ Insect repellent in the summer
- ➤ Maps or trail guides
- ➤ Pocketknife
- ➤ Raingear if rain is suspected
- ➤ Sunscreen
- ➤ Sunglasses
- ➤ Toilet paper or tissues and a plastic bag to hold soiled paper
- ➤ Water
- ➤ Whistle or pepper spray

If you're going on a long hike or bringing kids, consider toting a first aid kit:

➤ Antibiotic ointment

➤ Aspirin or acetaminophen

➤ Bandages

➤ Benadryl or the generic equivalent, diphenhydramine (*an antihistamine, in case of allergic reactions*)

➤ Elastic bandages or joint wraps

➤ Hydrogen peroxide or iodine

➤ Portable ice packs

➤ A prefilled syringe of epinephrine (*for those known to have severe allergic reactions to such things as bee stings*)

➤ Sunscreen

➤ Water-purification tablets or water filter (see note on page 6)

➤ Whistle (more effective in signaling rescuers than your voice)

Pack items in a waterproof bag or bags. Also, between hikes, remember to check expiration dates periodically. If you hike a lot, also think about taking a first aid class.

How to Deal with Potential Trail Hazards

It's easy to get into trouble when hiking. Here are some tips about taking care of yourself on the trail—in addition to making it a point to hike with at least one companion.

KNOW WHERE YOU ARE Guard against getting lost on the hike. Have a map and trail guide with you, along with a compass and/or GPS unit—and know how to use all of them. Try to keep track of where you are at all times. If you lose your way, the safest thing to do is retrace your steps. If backtracking gets you further lost, stop and seek help. Check a map. Watch for other hikers, or call for help on a cell phone, by using your whistle (three short blasts is the universal distress signal), or by yelling collectively with your companions. In general, you should stay put if it's getting dark.

WATCH YOUR STEP A common hiking hazard is tripping and falling down, thanks to rocks, tree roots, or uneven or slippery surfaces. Injury, especially to a lower limb, can take the fun out of any hike, so pay attention to comments about trail surfaces. Be smart on tricky trails, use caution when admiring a view, and watch where you put your feet.

GET OFF THE TRAIL BY DUSK Hiking after dark can be hazardous, so make sure you finish while there's still daylight. Take note of time estimates for each hike, and leave room for a margin of error. Keep a working flashlight in your pack.

AVOID POISON IVY AND STINGING NETTLES Poison ivy thrives throughout the area, in the city and in the countryside. It's both a climbing vine and a shrubby form of ground cover, identified by its telltale three leaflets to a leaf (hence the old adage "leaves of three, let it be"). Recognizing and avoiding contact with it is the most effective way to prevent the painful, oozing, and itchy rashes caused by urushiol, the oil in the plant's sap. Urushiol occurs in all parts of the plant (including the hairy vines that climb trees) and is active year-round. Raised lines and/or blisters, accompanied by itching, may appear within 48 hours of contact with the oil.

On exposure, flush the skin with water (or rub the area with wet mud, and then rinse). Then, when you can, wash the area with soap, dry it thoroughly, and, if a rash eventually appears, apply calamine lotion frequently to help dry it out. If itching or blistering is severe, seek medical attention. Also wash any urushiol-contaminated clothes or hiking gear. Remember that sensitivity to urushiol varies greatly from one person to the next, and that sensitivity tends to increase over time with repeated rash outbreaks.

Stinging nettles, with their typical serrate leaves, are a perennial that lines some trails during warm months. You'll remember them if your bare skin brushes against them, but the stinging doesn't last long for most people (minutes or hours, depending on individual sensitivity). The best prevention method is wearing long pants.

PROTECT YOURSELF AGAINST BITING AND STINGING INSECTS During the warm months in the Washington area, hikers are likely to be bugged mostly by mosquitoes, bees and wasps, ticks, and biting flies. There are also no-see-ums, chiggers, and even poisonous spiders, but they're rarely encountered. In all cases, though, practice prevention by using effective insect repellents and wearing long sleeves and pants with a tight weave.

Mosquitoes are the most common irritant, especially in the city itself and close-in urban areas, where the Asian tiger mosquito (*Aedes albopictus*) is an aggressive daytime biter. Local health authorities have also become concerned about the spread of the West Nile and Zika viruses by infected mosquitoes. However, there have been very few cases of West Nile and no cases of Zika in the area as of this writing. Nevertheless, health authorities recommend that people going outdoors take active measures to prevent getting bitten.

Bees and wasps, including hornets and yellow jackets, are occasionally aggressive, especially in the fall. Most people get stung when they venture too close to the underground lairs of yellow jackets. Be vigilant, and if you're highly allergic to bee or wasp stings (which can be fatal), be sure to carry an epinephrine-loaded syringe.

Ticks are also common and troublesome. They attach themselves to hikers who are walking through long grass, brushing past trailside bushes, or sitting on dead tree trunks. You won't feel them land on you or bite you, but it takes them a while to get settled on you and start feeding. In this area, the species of medical concern are the deer tick (about the size of the period at the end of this sentence), which may be infected with Lyme disease, and the dog tick (up to a half inch long), which may carry Rocky Mountain spotted fever. Insect repellents containing DEET are known to be effective deterrents. Most important, though, be sure to inspect yourself visually at the end of the hike; then later, while taking a shower, do a complete body check. For ticks that are already embedded, removal with tweezers is best. (To learn more about dealing with ticks, visit cdc.gov/ticks.)

STEER CLEAR OF ALL ANIMALS—AND HUNTERS The Washington area has a rich variety of animals, large and small, and hikers are usually thrilled to see most of them. However, give all animals you encounter a wide berth, both for their sake and yours. Although rarely dangerous, they can be a threat under certain circumstances, such as when surprised or cornered by humans. So be watchful, and do not, for example, get between a female bear and her cubs, try to pet a coyote, feed a deer, or approach a fox or raccoon during the day (they could be rabid).

Also stay away from all snakes. Only two poisonous ones inhabit the area— the timber rattlesnake and the copperhead—and neither is aggressive if left alone. Be careful where you put your hands and feet when crossing rocks or downed tree trunks, especially in late summer and early fall, when snakes seek out the sun.

During the hunting season, wear orange, be noisy, and avoid hunters in areas where hunting is allowed. If you feel uneasy, stay away altogether.

Hiking with Children

No one is too young for a nice hike in the woods or through a city park. Parents can carry infants and toddlers in special carriers. Older children, of course, can follow along with adults. Use common sense to judge a child's capability, endurance, and attention span. When packing for the hike, remember the children's needs as well as your own. Make sure they wear adequate clothing and shoes for the weather, and remember that they dehydrate quickly. Kids don't know when they've developed a blister, so stop and check their feet periodically. We designed this book to be family friendly and believe that most children can do the shorter hikes in this book.

The Flora and Fauna of the Mid-Atlantic

SPECIES YOU MAY FIND ON THESE HIKES

Throughout this book, we mention names of plants and wildlife you might encounter. Some park environments are rich in diverse vegetation and provide idyllic

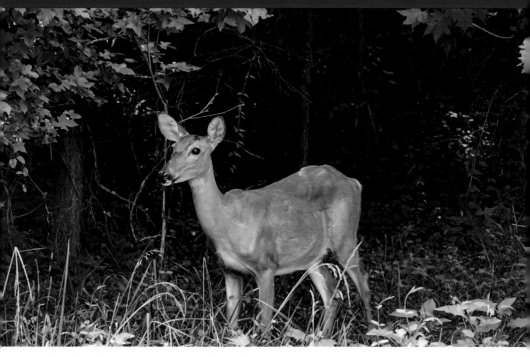

White-tailed deer are common in D.C.'s urban parks.

woodland habitats for birds, reptiles, and mammals. Often parklands have been set aside to preserve native species.

The mid-Atlantic region has a wide array of charming critters. Black squirrels are seen quite often here. White-tailed deer are ubiquitous in our urban parks. Our proximity to the Chesapeake Bay, Anacostia River, and Potomac River makes this the home of a diverse population of animal life and more than 240 species of birds. But keep in mind, the wildlife you see on your hike is determined by weather, time of day, and how busy the park is.

The goal of the park's custodians is to protect natural spaces and native plants and animals from the threat of development. But you'll find that many of these parks, especially those in the national parks system, are crowded on weekends and holidays. That's why we recommend visiting on weekdays, when possible, or early in the morning on weekends. Winter is a quiet time in parks, and that's also when it's easier to spot wildlife, especially birds.

INVASIVE SPECIES

According to the Potomac Conservancy, the Chesapeake Bay watershed loses an estimated 70 acres of forest land each day. As the human population encroaches on natural habitats and international trade introduces new species to the environment, native plants and animals come under siege. Invasive vines, such as kudzu and English ivy, are strangling trees and shrubs, and local deer, with few natural predators, have become overpopulated. Because they consume massive amounts of vegetation, they are destroying the natural habitat of other wildlife. Native plants and animals possess natural defenses against insects and diseases but struggle to compete with invasive species. A balance is difficult to achieve. If you want to learn more about these issues, consult the Sierra Club, Audubon Society, Potomac Conservancy, or National Park Service National Capital Region. Volunteer groups lead efforts to clear invasive plants and educate the community on the best practices for protecting our natural resources.

COMMONLY SEEN WILDLIFE AND VEGETATION

What might you see in the wilds around Washington, D.C.? There are more than 1,000 plant species found in northern Virginia, the District of Columbia, and Maryland. Under the heading of botanical, there are flowering and nonflowering plants, algae, lichens, and mushrooms. The most commonly found trees in our local forests are deciduous, although there are multiple variations of evergreen and conifer trees too. Although some plants are edible, we don't recommend you sample any. Of the hundreds of mushroom species in the region, at least 10 are poisonous.

Commonly seen trees in the mid-Atlantic are the papaw, persimmon, Eastern white pine, loblolly pine, redbud, and sassafras. Some have showy flowers, such as the Southern magnolia, or fruits, such as the American holly. The largest, widest trees are often hardwoods such as red and sugar maple, river birch, hickory, black walnut, sweet gum, and multiple oaks, including post, swamp, white, scarlet, pin, willow, and red. Notice those trees with the white bark growing along the shoreline of the Potomac River? They are sycamores. Sadly, many of the magnificent American elms that once shaded the National Mall have succumbed to Dutch elm disease.

Also in the mid-Atlantic are thriving populations of foxes, hares, squirrels, bats, groundhogs and chipmunks. You probably won't see them, but there are owls, beavers, mice, muskrats, opossums, otters, raccoons, skunks, and weasels living in the wild. The parks in this book

One of hiking's greatest rewards is observing the many bird species that thrive in these protected landscapes.

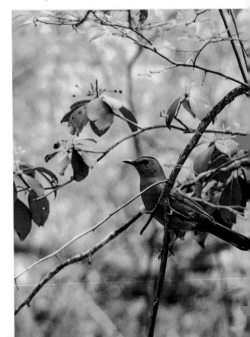

have played an integral role in the rejuvenation of the bald eagle and wild turkey populations. Keep a lookout for Canada geese, vultures, songbirds, and reptiles in the woodlands and wetlands.

CITY OF TREES

Author Melanie Choukas Bradley, vice president of the Maryland Native Plant Society, gave Washington, D.C., the moniker City of Trees in her 2008 book *City of Trees: The Complete Guide to the Trees of Washington, D.C.* The guide identifies more than 300 species of trees and documents the efforts of prominent Washingtonians to plant and preserve the city's urban tree canopy. In 2012 the city's urban canopy had grown by 2.1%, covering nearly 38% of the city (determined using aerial data). One of the many reasons hiking here is particularly interesting is seeing our trees change with the seasons. During the winter, when the leaves have fallen, the views and vistas are wide open. Spring is our most beloved season, thanks to the famous cherry blossom trees and others that flower before producing leaves. Autumn brings a riot of color to our parks. As days grow shorter and the growing season ends, deciduous trees end the daily process of photosynthesis, which turns leaves green. After the bright green fades away, it is replaced with yellows and reds. Because of the region's impressive foliage, along with cooling temperatures, fall is probably the local hiker's favorite season.

Hikers follow the stone path across a creek at Prince William Forest Park (Hike 59, page 270).

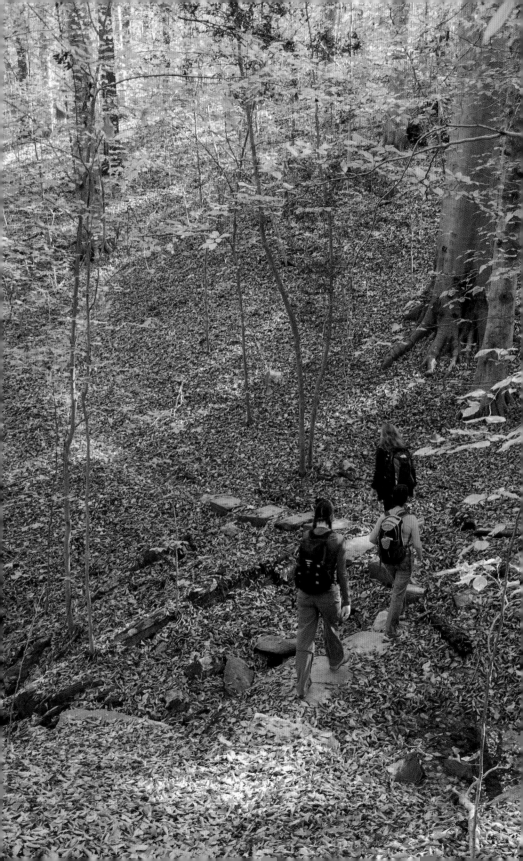

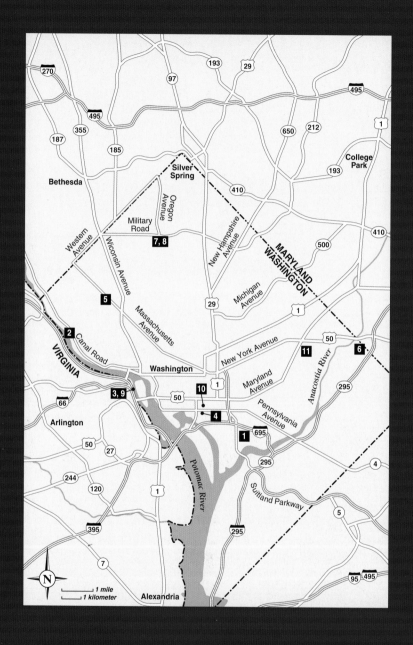

WASHINGTON, D.C.

1 ANACOSTIA RIVERWALK TRAIL

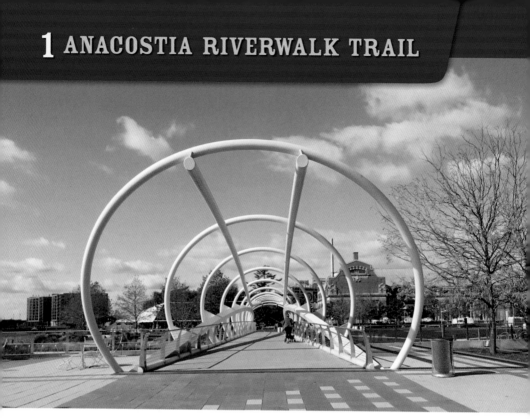

The bridge at Yards Parks runs over the Anacostia Riverwalk Trail connecting Nationals Park with the Capitol Riverfront neighborhood.

THIS IS AN URBAN WALK with panoramic views of the Anacostia River and the Washington Navy Yard, plus other points of interest along the way. The trail is easy to reach by Metro.

DESCRIPTION

The Anacostia Riverwalk is a 20-mile multiuse trail that is under construction along the east and west banks of the Anacostia River, stretching from Prince George's County in Maryland to Washington, D.C. Twelve miles of the trail were complete as of mid-2017. When the trail is finished, it will provide a scenic route for pedestrians and bicyclists along the river to the Fish Market, Nationals Park, Historic Anacostia, RFK Stadium, the National Arboretum, and 16 communities between the National Mall at the Tidal Basin and Bladensburg Marina Park in Maryland.

This walk begins at the Navy Yard Metro station at the corner of M Street Southeast and New Jersey Avenue. When you exit the Metro station, be sure to follow the signs to the New Jersey Avenue exit. If you choose to drive, park at one of the paid parking garages, and find your way to this intersection. Follow New Jersey Avenue toward the waterfront.

LENGTH 2.1 miles (with longer options)

CONFIGURATION Out-and-back

DIFFICULTY Easy

SCENERY Cityscapes, river views

EXPOSURE Open

TRAFFIC Light; moderate–heavy on warm-weather evenings, weekends, and holidays

TRAIL SURFACE Boardwalk and pavement

HIKING TIME 1–1.5 hours

DRIVING DISTANCE 1.4 miles

SEASON Year-round

ACCESS The area in front of the Navy Yard is open daily from sunrise to 2 hours after sunset, although it is sometimes closed for events that require security.

WHEELCHAIR TRAVERSABLE Yes

MAPS Anacostia Waterfront Initiative, anacostiawaterfront.org/resources/maps

FACILITIES Restrooms at restaurants in the area

CONTACT Anacostia Waterfront Initiative, anacostiawaterfront.org, Capitol Riverfront Business Improvement District (BID), capitol riverfront.org

LOCATION Yards Park and Capitol Riverfront, Washington, D.C.

COMMENTS The Riverwalk Trail will eventually link to more than 40 miles of trails in Maryland. This short section provides great recreational opportunities in a growing area of the city but at the time of this writing does not yet connect to the rest of the trail.

On your left, you will see the headquarters for the U.S. Department of Transportation. At the far end of the building, turn left onto the Transportation Walk, which is an outdoor museum that explores the history of transportation with interpretive panels and life-size elements of transportation. When you reach Third Street, turn right and continue toward the waterfront.

At Water Street, the dancing water fountain at the entrance to Yards Park provides a splashing and cooling-off venue for families during the summer months. Go to the right of the fountain and take the steps down; then follow the path to the right, and turn left to cross over the riverfront boardwalk and 200-foot steel pedestrian bridge. Swing to the left and follow the path along the waterfront, turning right and then left again to connect to the Anacostia Riverwalk Trail. Enjoy the views of the River Street Gardens to your left. River birches shade small seating areas furnished with benches that face the river. Turn around and look behind the Yards Park Bridge for a view of Nationals Park, Washington's baseball stadium. Continue east; the views of the Anacostia are delightful on a sunny day.

As you walk along the trail, you will cross through an entrance to the walkway in front of the Washington Navy Yard. The facility is heavily guarded and has a high iron-rod fence. You cannot enter the Navy Yard without an appropriate ID and/or an escort. As you reach the far end of the trail, stop to visit a display of the Vietnam War swift boat, a US Navy vessel used in coastal and river operations to search for North Vietnamese steel-hulled ships, junks, and other craft attempting to deliver arms and munitions to enemy forces ashore.

Anacostia Riverwalk Trail

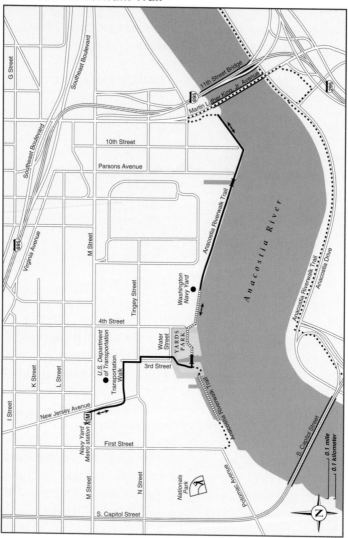

As you exit the Navy Yard area, you can turn left to follow the path toward Capitol Hill (about a mile's walk to Eastern Market) or turn around to return to Yards Park. The Anacostia Riverwalk trail will eventually cross the 11th Street Bridge and continue farther east.

The 11th Street Bridge connects Washington, D.C.'s Capitol Hill and Anacostia neighborhoods and is slated to become the city's first elevated park, a one-of-a-kind civic space that is being compared to New York City's High Line. The new bridge will provide a venue for recreation, environmental education, and the arts and will be designed to include performance spaces, playgrounds, and classrooms. The 11th Street Bridge/Park is projected to open in mid-2019.

NEARBY/RELATED ACTIVITIES

Check out the restaurants in the Capitol Riverfront neighborhood. Attend a baseball game at Nationals Park (mlb.com/nationals) or attend a festival at the Yards (theyards dc.com). Explore the Navy Museum (history.navy.mil) and the Navy Art Gallery (tinyurl.com/navyartcoll) to learn about the Navy's history from the Revolutionary War to the present. In winter, go ice skating at Canal Park (capitolriverfront.org).

• •

GPS TRAILHEAD COORDINATES N38° 52.592' W77° 0.257'

DIRECTIONS From Exit 43 on the Capital Beltway (I-495), take the George Washington Memorial Parkway to the I-395 North/14th Street Bridge. At the end of the bridge, I-395 branches right and becomes the Southeast–Southwest Freeway. Take the freeway to the Sixth Street Southeast exit. The sign also says Navy Yard. Proceed down the ramp and continue straight to Eighth Street; turn right on Eighth Street, then right onto M Street. Street parking is very limited in the area. Park in a paid garage near Nationals Park.

The paved trail along the Capitol Riverfront offers scenic views of Nationals Park and the Anacostia River.

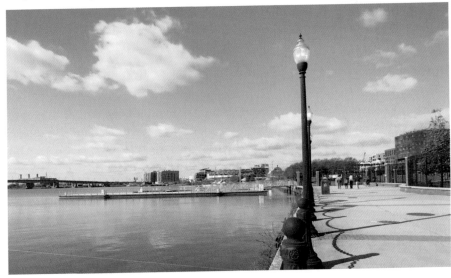

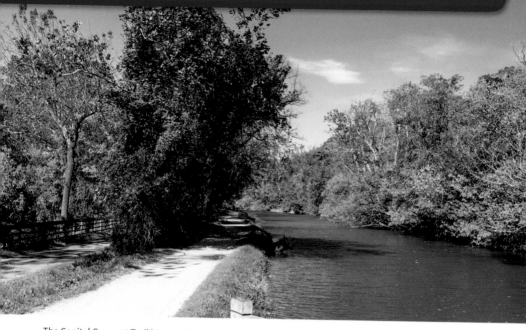

The Capital Crescent Trail is a scenic path that runs parallel to the C&O Canal and its towpath.

A FORMER RAILROAD RIGHT-OF-WAY, the multiuse trail curves through close-in suburban Maryland and Northwest Washington. Its paved lower segment provides hikers with a good workout and scenic outing in a parkland setting. The 10-acre Georgetown Waterfront Park offers visitors a place to enjoy river views at the edge of a historic urban neighborhood.

DESCRIPTION

The Capital Crescent Trail (CCT) is a narrow, parkland-encased pathway that arcs smoothly through affluent neighborhoods for 11 miles between Maryland's Silver Spring and Washington's Georgetown waterfront. The country's most used rail trail, it has been heralded by the International Project for Public Places as one of the world's "21 great places that show how transportation can enliven a community."

   The trail's lower and paved segment that starts at Fletcher's Cove is popular year-round, mostly as a neighborhood recreational destination. Fletcher's Boathouse is a National Park Service concession that is open early March–October and rents rowboats, kayaks, canoes, and bicycles. Across the towpath from Fletcher's is the Abner Cloud House. It is the oldest structure on the C&O Canal, built in the early 1800s. The house was a residence and storeroom for the grains shipped to Georgetown.

LENGTH 5.5 miles (with shorter and longer options)

CONFIGURATION Out-and-back

DIFFICULTY Easy

SCENERY Cityscapes, river views

EXPOSURE Shady; less so in winter

TRAFFIC Moderate–heavy, especially on warm-weather evenings, weekends, and holidays

TRAIL SURFACE Paved

HIKING TIME 2.5 hours

DRIVING DISTANCE 6.6 miles

SEASON Year-round

ACCESS No restrictions

WHEELCHAIR TRAVERSABLE Yes

MAPS Coalition for the Capital Crescent Trail, cctrail.org/maps; Montgomery Parks, montgomeryparks.org

FACILITIES Restrooms at trailhead and at restaurants in Georgetown

CONTACT Coalition for the Capital Crescent Trail, cctrail.org; Friends of Georgetown Waterfront Park, georgetownwaterfrontpark.org

LOCATION Northwest Washington, D.C.

COMMENTS The trail is very flat and popular for walking, jogging, biking, and in-line skating. Although you can access the Capital Crescent Trail (CCT) from multiple points, this 5.5-mile section is the most scenic. You can walk in the reverse direction by starting in Georgetown. Stay to your right and avoid speeding cyclists and in-line skaters.

It may seem a bit odd that a trail completed in 1996 can go right through such a built-over and pricey area, as well as downtown Bethesda. The explanation is that, although the CCT itself is new, the route is more than a century old and predates modern suburban expansion. For much of the 20th century, it was the right-of-way of a railroad spur line that delivered coal and building supplies to the industry-cluttered Georgetown waterfront. That fact also explains the route's gentle grades, with only 350 feet of elevation change between Georgetown and Bethesda. When its last coal customer switched to truck delivery in 1985, the rail line was closed.

The following year, volunteers organized the Coalition for the Capital Crescent Trail to campaign for converting the private right-of-way into a public, multiuse trail. With the help of assorted organizations, public agencies, individuals, and good luck, the effort succeeded. Today, the Washington, D.C., portion of the CCT is managed by the National Park Service as part of the adjoining Chesapeake & Ohio Canal National Historical Park. The Maryland portion is owned and maintained by Montgomery County.

Now a thriving membership organization, the Coalition for the Capital Crescent Trail continues to press for completion of the 4-mile section between Bethesda and Silver Spring. That section, called the Georgetown Branch Trail, is passable but currently is only a crushed-stone "interim trail" with on-street detours. Although the section is a key link to trails in and beyond Maryland's Rock Creek Regional Park, various political and funding issues continue to complicate its completion.

To get started from the parking lot at Fletcher's, head downriver on the paved CCT (rather than the adjoining dirt-surfaced C&O Canal towpath), keeping the Potomac River to your right. You won't see much of the river for about a mile, thanks

Capital Crescent Trail: Fletcher's Cove to Georgetown Waterfront Park

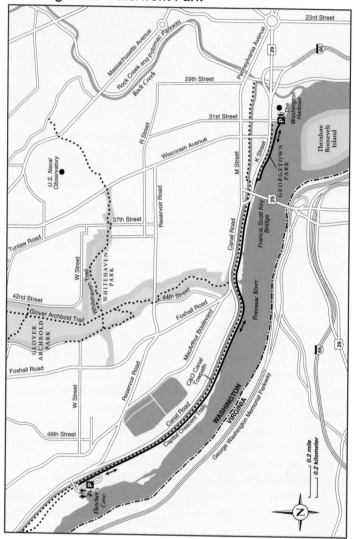

to the thickly wooded floodplain. As you reach downtown, watch for kayakers and sculling teams along the water. As you pass by the Washington Canoe Club and approach Francis Scott Key Bridge, the trail ends. Continue walking along K Street (carefully avoiding traffic), and then turn right into Georgetown Waterfront Park. Then turn left and walk along the Potomac waterfront. Enjoy views of Key Bridge; the Rosslyn, Virginia, skyline; the John F. Kennedy Center for the Performing Arts;

and Theodore Roosevelt Island. The park was completed in 2011 and features walk-ways, benches, a large fountain, and scenic overlooks with granite slabs etched with scenes from the waterfront's history as a seaport. The steps are a prime place for pic-nicking, watching shorebirds, or viewing paddlers on the river. If you keep walking to the far end of the park, you will reach Washington Harbour, a multipurpose prop-erty that features luxury condominiums, office space, a public boardwalk, and sev-eral restaurants that offer alfresco dining. After eating, resting, or exploring awhile, retrace your steps 3.3 miles back to Fletcher's Cove.

NEARBY/RELATED ACTIVITIES

Explore the river or canal in a Fletcher's rental boat (202-337-9642, boatingindc .com; available during warm-weather months), or picnic at Fletcher's spacious riverside park. Allow time to visit Georgetown, where you can shop, dine, or visit a wide range of attractions. Visit the National Park Service Visitor Center along the C&O Canal at 1057 Thomas Jefferson St. NW, Washington, D.C. (accessible from 30th Street).

· ·

GPS TRAILHEAD COORDINATES N38° 55.149' W77° 06.093'

DIRECTIONS From the Capital Beltway (I-495), take the Glen Echo exit (Exit 41) onto Clara Barton Parkway. Follow Clara Barton Parkway until it becomes Canal Road (at Chain Bridge). Continue on Canal Road until the entrance of Fletcher's at Canal and Reservoir. Fletcher's is located on the right side of the road next to the canal. The entrance is a 180-degree turn, and there is not enough room to maneuver. You cannot access the area southbound on Canal Road. From this direction, you have to pass the entrance and make a U-turn.

From the Georgetown end of Key Bridge in Northwest Washington, drive west on M Street Northwest/Canal Road 0.5 mile. At the third traffic light, turn left to stay on Canal Road. Go 1.6 miles to Fletcher's Boathouse, on the left.

Parking is available on both sides of the canal at Fletcher's Cove—near the entrance next to the historic Abner Cloud House and near the Potomac, next to the boathouse. To get to the Potomac-area parking lot, drive through the tunnel that crosses the canal.

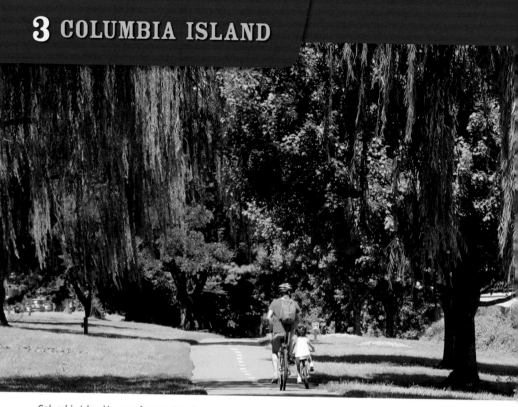

Columbia Island is one of many sites that run along the Mount Vernon Trail, a multiuse recreation trail that parallels the George Washington Memorial Parkway.

BEGINNING AT THEODORE ROOSEVELT ISLAND, this hike is a modified loop to maximize views and stops at points of interest along Columbia Island. Hidden in plain sight, the island lies on the Potomac River across from the Lincoln Memorial. Often mistaken for part of Virginia, it offers sweeping views of some of Washington's most iconic landmarks.

DESCRIPTION

Columbia Island came to be in 1916, when the Potomac River was dredged and the spoils were piled up on the Virginia shore. Because the new land formed an island, it automatically became part of Washington, D.C., thanks to an ancient law denying Virginia even part ownership of the Potomac. But that didn't prevent Virginia from protesting. The matter was settled in the 1930s, when the District received the island and Virginia received reclaimed land later developed as Reagan National Airport. That same decade, the island became a key link in the metro area's growing road network. The island was also landscaped, but its primary purpose was to carry motor traffic.

In 1968 the National Park Service designated the 121-acre island as Lady Bird Johnson Park to honor the then–First Lady's efforts to beautify the country. The Lyndon Baines Johnson Memorial Grove was added in 1974, the year after the

LENGTH 4.5 miles

CONFIGURATION Modified loop

DIFFICULTY Easy

SCENERY Waterside parklands, cross-Potomac views of mainland Washington

EXPOSURE Mostly open

TRAFFIC Generally light; moderate on Mount Vernon Trail on warm-weather evenings, weekends, and holidays

TRAIL SURFACE Mostly pavement and boardwalk; some grass and dirt

HIKING TIME 2–2.5 hours

DRIVING DISTANCE 4.5 miles

SEASON Year-round

ACCESS Mount Vernon Trail closes at dark.

WHEELCHAIR TRAVERSABLE No

MAP USGS *Washington West*

FACILITIES Restrooms, water, phones, and café at marina; water at LBJ Memorial Grove

CONTACT George Washington Memorial Parkway, 703-289-2500 or nps.gov/gwmp

LOCATION Arlington, Virginia

COMMENTS The hike involves crossing the George Washington Memorial Parkway and a short jaunt along the busy roadway. Be very careful when crossing roads; the best and safest time to do this hike is on weekday afternoons or weekend mornings. To shorten the hike and avoid crossing roads, stay on the Mount Vernon Trail and retrace your steps in an out-and-back excursion.

ex-president died. The island now has many dogwoods, pines, and flowering bushes, as well as myriad daffodils and fine views of mainland Washington and the river.

This hike is a 4.5-mile counterclockwise loop that follows much of the perimeter of the mostly flat island. It crosses heavily traveled and high-speed roadways, so be vigilant.

Starting from the parking-lot trailhead at Theodore Roosevelt Island, march to the lot's south end, and proceed on the mostly paved Mount Vernon Trail. At the first T junction, turn left to stay close to the river, following the signage toward Reagan National Airport and Mount Vernon. Walk over the wooden boardwalk that runs along the Potomac River, passing large weeping willow trees and sweeping views of the Washington Monument, Lincoln Memorial, and Kennedy Center. About 50 yards before reaching the Memorial Bridge, turn right and follow the small trail through the grass to climb the slope toward George Washington Memorial Parkway. Look left to watch for traffic, and carefully cross the road. Cross a second time, and then follow the sidewalk to the right to cross the crosswalk for a third time. Follow the sidewalk to the far side of the circle, crossing the road to pass the entrance to Arlington National Cemetery.

Continue on the grass south toward Reagan National Airport until you see the walking path to your left. Cross the road to reach the paved path toward the Pentagon. At the parking lot, continue straight, and look for the stairs and bridge that crosses over the Boundary Channel. Cross to the center of the 15-acre Lyndon B. Johnson Memorial Grove. There, set on a circular paving-stone plaza rimmed with

Columbia Island

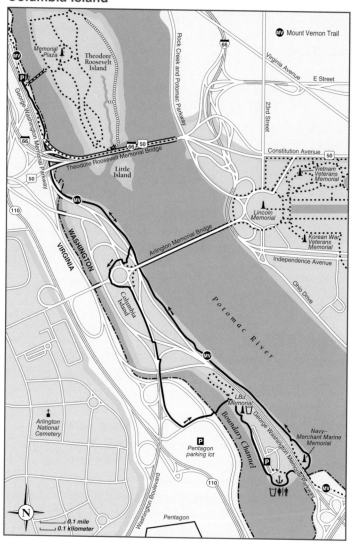

white pines, is a rough-hewn, 19-foot-high slab of granite from Texas (President Johnson's home state). Retrace your steps on the flagstone path to the first junction. There, turn left onto a gravel path; then go right at the next fork and walk through Columbia Island marina's parking lot to the café's patio. Cross over the grass toward the paved path, and walk underneath the bridge back toward the Potomac River. You will come to the Navy–Merchant Marine Memorial on your left, with its seven aluminum seagulls skimming the crest of a large aluminum wave breaking across a granite base. Then follow the Mount Vernon Trail north, and hike 2 miles back to the trailhead, keeping right at each intersection.

NEARBY/RELATED ACTIVITIES

For a glorious postscript, do the 2-mile circuit around Roosevelt Island (Hike 9, page 52), or cross the Arlington Memorial Bridge and do the Tidal Basin and West Potomac Park hike (Hike 10, page 57). There are multiple places to dine and shop in nearby Crystal City and Rosslyn. Or visit Old Town Alexandria and take a boat ride up the Potomac.

· ·

GPS TRAILHEAD COORDINATES N38° 53.738' W77° 04.001'

DIRECTIONS Theodore Roosevelt Island is accessible only from the northbound lanes of the George Washington Memorial Parkway. The entrance to the parking lot is located just north of the Roosevelt Bridge.

From Exit 43 on the Capital Beltway, take George Washington Memorial Parkway south toward Washington, D.C. Pass Roosevelt Island, and exit toward Memorial Bridge. At the traffic circle, take the second exit onto South Arlington Boulevard. Use the right two lanes to take the ramp to I-66/I-495/Spout Run Parkway/McLean. Merge onto the GW Parkway. Take the first exit into the Theodore Roosevelt Island parking lot on the right.

The Navy–Merchant Marine Memorial, located in Lady Bird Johnson Park on Columbia Island, honors sailors who died at sea during World War I.

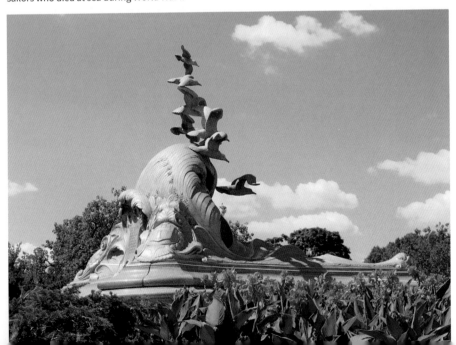

From the National Mall area, head west on Constitution Avenue to cross Theodore Roosevelt Memorial Bridge, staying to the right. Take the first exit to the right and then another right onto northbound George Washington Memorial Parkway. Take the first exit (within 300 yards) into Theodore Roosevelt Island parking lot on the right. To get there from the parkway's southbound lanes, cross into Washington, turn around, and follow the directions above. Note: To return to Washington or the southbound lanes after your hike, drive north on the parkway 0.7 mile, and take the first exit on the left onto Spout Run Parkway. Then either take the first exit on the left to get onto the southbound parkway, or continue to Lee Highway, which connects to local streets and I-66.

Or take the Metro and walk to the trailhead. Take the Orange or Blue Line train to Rosslyn Metro station, and then walk 0.8 mile to the trailhead: From the station's main entrance, turn left and walk north (downhill) on North Moore Street, cross North 19th Street, turn right alongside Lee Highway, cross North Lynn Street, turn left and walk north on North Lynn, and cross Lee Highway. At the far corner, turn right onto the signposted Mount Vernon Trail, and follow it to the trailhead. Contact Metro, 202-637-7000 or wmata.com.

Columbia Island Marina on the Potomac River has a prime location off the George Washington Memorial Parkway and provides slips and services for boaters.

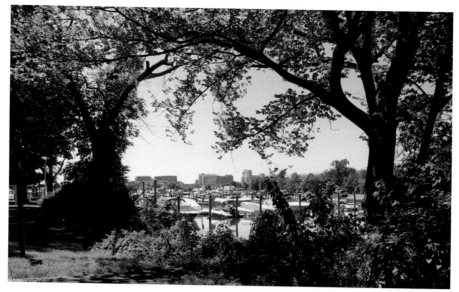

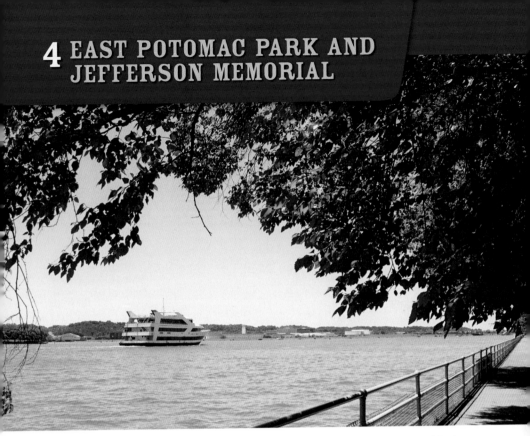

From East Potomac Park, you'll see tour boats leaving from Gangplank Marina and The Wharf; both are located across the Washington Channel from East Potomac Park.

EXTENDING SOUTH FROM THE MALL, Potomac Park is just the place for a hike that features waterfront views of southwest Washington and northern Virginia, the Tidal Basin, memorials, golf and tennis courts, and much open space.

DESCRIPTION

Potomac Park is one of the youngest parks in Washington, dating from the 1880s. Located on a spit of land between the Washington Channel and the Potomac River, the park features an abundance of free and inexpensive recreational facilities operated by the National Park Service. Tennis, golf, swimming, minigolf, and picnicking are popular activities here, but the park is also a favorite with local fishermen. The path is flooded fairly frequently, but fortunately there's plenty of space to detour around the puddles.

Our 6.1-mile loop hike begins on the National Mall and hugs the shoreline of East Potomac Park. Start from the Smithsonian Metro station, walking toward the Department of Agriculture building on Independence Avenue and 12th Street. Walk past the Capital BikeShare kiosk toward C Street. Cross C Street and then turn right

29

LENGTH 6.1 miles

CONFIGURATION Loop

DIFFICULTY Easy–moderate

SCENERY Parklands, waterfront views, street scenes

EXPOSURE Mostly open

TRAFFIC In Tidal Basin area, moderate–heavy in cherry-blossom season, especially on weekends and holidays; lighter at other times. Elsewhere, light year-round.

TRAIL SURFACE Pavement

HIKING TIME 2.5 hours

DRIVING DISTANCE 3 miles

SEASON Year-round, but best in cooler weather

ACCESS No restrictions

WHEELCHAIR TRAVERSABLE Some paved roads, but sidewalks are torn up in many places

MAPS USGS *Washington West*; ADC *Metro Washington*

FACILITIES Restrooms at museums and hotels; water and food in Mall museums

CONTACT National Capital Parks—Central, 202-619-7222 or nps.gov/nacc; Cultural Tourism DC, culturaltourismdc.org

LOCATION Washington, D.C.

COMMENTS Finish this hike by sunset.

on D Street, continuing past 13th Street. To your left, you'll see the Mandarin Oriental hotel and catch a glimpse of the Jefferson Memorial.

Walk to the bottom of the hill on a road paralleling 14th Street. You'll pass parking lots and arrive at the busy and complicated intersection of Maine Avenue, Martin Luther King Jr. Avenue, and 14th Street. To your left you'll see The Wharf and Maine Avenue Fish Market, which is a fun place to explore and pick up some refreshments for the hike.

Cross underneath the multiple overpasses here, ending up on the walkway by MLK Avenue. Proceed to the crosswalk and carefully cross MLK Avenue and Ohio Drive. In front of you is the Jefferson Memorial; to the right, the Tidal Basin.

Walk a few yards on the paved path that flanks the Tidal Basin, and you'll be walking through a man-made landscape. The land itself did not exist until the 1880s. Back then, the area consisted of often-flooded swamplands and mudflats along the silted-up Potomac River. Then came Peter Hains, an Army officer who happened to be between wars (a Civil War veteran, he later served in both the Spanish-American War and World War I). To build up the mudflats and make the river more navigable, he ordered the dredging of the river's main channel and Washington Channel, with the spoils to be piled between them. Held in place by a seawall, the spoils formed a long, uvula-like peninsula.

The Tidal Basin was created in the following decade. It was built to collect river water to be released into the pier-lined Washington Channel when water levels got too low. Subsequently, the new lands were landscaped. In 1912, 3,000 flowering cherry trees—a gift from Japan to the United States—were planted around the

East Potomac Park and Jefferson Memorial

Tidal Basin (today, only about 100 survive; the rest are replacements). Starting in the 1920s the basin also served as a whites-only public swimming pool, complete with a sandy beach, and the federal government operated a 60-acre tourist camp for visiting motorists on the peninsula. The resort disappeared with the construction of the Jefferson Memorial, which opened in 1943. Today, the Tidal Basin and the adjoining areas that make up West Potomac Park are a world-famous tourist attraction, and in spring the basin's walkways are wreathed in cherry blossoms and upturned faces.

At the Jefferson Memorial, pause to take in views of the nearby Franklin D. Roosevelt Memorial (see Hike 10, page 57) and Martin Luther King Jr. Memorial (in the distance). If you are so inclined, step in to see the statue of Thomas Jefferson and read the wall panels of quotes by the Founding Father, including parts of the Declaration of Independence. Then resume walking west toward the junction of East Basin Drive and Ohio Drive. Cross Ohio Drive carefully, following the sign pointing to East Potomac Park (the sign also indicates the locations of West Potomac Park, Southwest Waterfront, and Nationals Park).

You'll cross under an overpass by Memorial Park's headquarters on the left to enter East Potomac Park. Begin your hike on the paved perimeter path that will be your route for the next 4 miles, offering views of the Washington Marina, Fort McNair, and The Wharf across the Washington Channel. Due to funding challenges, Potomac Park is not well maintained, so beware of loose concrete and deep holes.

As you're walking, keep an eye out for the water taxis and sightseeing boats that begin in the Washington Channel heading in and out of the Potomac River. Continuing, you'll reach Hains Point, a windy but bird-rich, open spot where the Anacostia River joins the Potomac. Pause to appreciate the panoramic views.

Stay on the sidewalk as it swings right for your first views of Alexandria, Reagan National Airport, Crystal City, and the Woodrow Wilson Bridge. Look back up the Potomac to see Georgetown University and the National Cathedral in the distance.

The walk proceeds along the Potomac River, heading northwest and back to the entrance of the park. Pass the U.S. Park Police offices on the left, and follow signs back to the National Mall by retracing your steps to the Smithsonian Metro station.

NEARBY/RELATED ACTIVITIES

Across the Washington Channel is the new Wharf development. This mile-long stretch along the Potomac River has restaurants, shops, residences, and office space, all with views of the marinas, Theodore Roosevelt Island, and the river. Stop at the historic Maine Avenue Fish Market or catch some music at one of the Wharf's new venues. For details, call 202-688-3590 or visit wharfdc.com.

• •

GPS TRAILHEAD COORDINATES N38° 53.254' W77° 01.694'

DIRECTIONS Head for the Mall area. If you wish to drive, look for parking near L'Enfant Plaza or C Street, or at the Tidal Basin Paddle Boats parking lot. It's best to arrive early on crowded warm-weather weekends and holidays; heed local parking regulations (read signs carefully). Or use the Metro: Smithsonian station is on the Orange and Blue lines; Metrobuses operate on nearby streets. Contact Metro, 202-637-7000 or wmata.com.

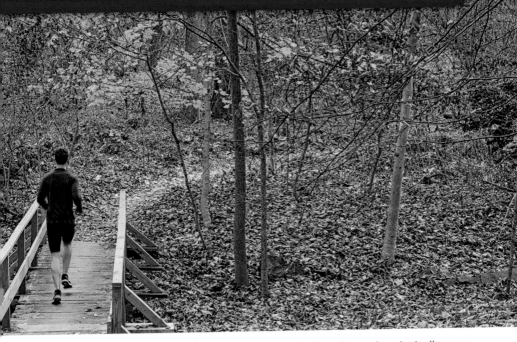

Glover Archbold Park offers a scenic, wooded path that is popular for walking and running in all seasons.

HIKERS MAKE THEIR WAY through the heavily wooded stream valley of Glover Archbold Park from American University to the C&O Canal surrounded by upscale neighborhoods in Northwest Washington.

DESCRIPTION

Glover Archbold Park is an urban oasis with a unique combination of residential, historical, and commercial enterprises existing harmoniously in a natural sanctuary. It's popular with city dwellers, who use it to run, hike, and walk their dogs. Protected by the National Park Service and part of the Potomac Heritage Trail Network, this trail starts and ends on Massachusetts Avenue Northwest, meandering through hilly woodlands and crossing three roadways. The landscape was created through man-made and natural developments, including a dam and erosion from Foundry Branch. Called the Lafayette Plateau, the mounds of gray-blue stone (known as Kensington granite) are up to 50 feet high on either side of the trail.

Charles Glover, the president of Riggs Bank, and Anne Mills Archbold, daughter of John Archbold, whose oil company merged with Standard Oil Trust, donated land to create their namesake park. Between 1923 and 1933, the two philanthropists led

LENGTH 4.8 miles (with longer options)

CONFIGURATION Out-and-back

DIFFICULTY Easy–moderate

SCENERY Woodlands, river views, street scenes, stream valley

EXPOSURE Mostly shady; less so in winter

TRAFFIC Moderate; heavy on warm-weather evenings, weekends, and holidays

TRAIL SURFACE Mostly dirt; some pavement

HIKING TIME 2 hours

DRIVING DISTANCE 7 miles

SEASON Year-round

ACCESS Trails open daily, sunrise–sunset

WHEELCHAIR TRAVERSABLE No

MAPS None

FACILITIES None

CONTACT Potomac Heritage National Scenic Trail office, 304-535-4014, nps.gov/pohe

LOCATION Northwest Washington, D.C.

COMMENTS On Massachusetts Avenue, there is free parking without meters, except for rush hour (7–10 a.m.) on weekdays. You can also take a bus from the Tenleytown Metro station to the trailhead.

efforts to preserve scenic and recreational opportunities in a city that was expanding quickly. Years later, environmentalist Rachel Carson took a well-publicized walk in the park, drawing attention to the importance of their preservation efforts.

The trail begins on Massachusetts Avenue, about 0.5 mile southeast of Nebraska Avenue, between the soaring high-rise condominiums that make up the American University Park and Cathedral Heights neighborhoods. Look for the sign to Glover Archbold Park and descend wooden railroad ties to the valley below.

Follow the yellow blazes past a redbrick high-rise and a concrete structure decorated with graffiti. Next pass an open concrete pipe used by the D.C. water and sewer service. The Northwest D.C. sewer-shed flows through Glover Archbold Park, consisting of manholes and pipelines constructed in the early 20th century. At nearly 100 years old, the pipes have reached their maximum expected life span; the water and sewer authority is in the process of rehabilitating the aging sewer infrastructure.

Along this trail are several stream bridges and sewer caps. You'll remain in the forested valley until you come to Cathedral Avenue. Use the crosswalk and continue down the steps on Glover Archbold Trail. Cross New Mexico Avenue/Tunlaw Road and pick up the trail to the left (on Garfield Street). Stop to read the sign detailing the park's history. It was installed by the National Park Service on the 54th anniversary of the publication of Rachel Carson's book *Silent Spring*.

After walking through an open meadow, cross a small wooden bridge over Foundry Stream. Look to your left to see the Glover Park Community Garden, where local residents can rent a small plot of land to grow their own produce. Then the trail continues a short distance over an exposed concrete sewer pipe.

Glover Archbold Park Trail intersects two other trails during this hike. First is the Wesley Heights Trail that leads to Foxhall Road and the Battery-Kemble Trail. If

Glover Archbold Park Trail and Potomac Heritage Trail

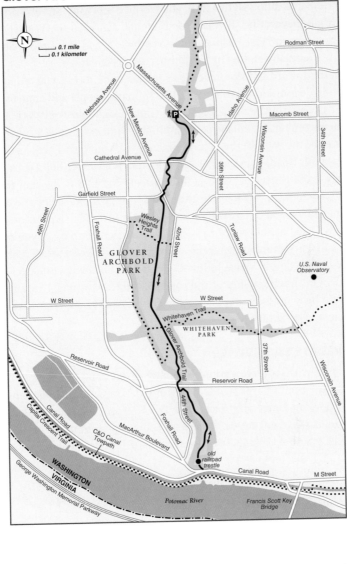

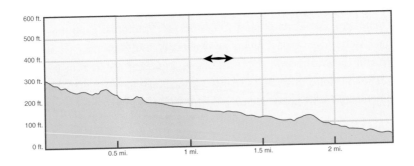

you turned right and followed this trail, you would come to W Street Northwest and pass the Foxhall Playground. If you turned left and followed the Whitehaven Trail, it would bring you to Wisconsin Avenue Northwest, and the United States Naval Observatory, eventually ending up in Dumbarton Oaks Park.

Continuing toward the Potomac River in this thick forest, you're likely to pass herds of gentle deer or kids netting tadpoles. So many people and animals enjoy this refuge, you can't help but be thankful that the Glover Archbold Trail was rescued again in 1962 from becoming a multilane parkway. In the winter when the leaves have fallen, you might notice the walls of the French Embassy on your left. Then, just before you come to Reservoir Road, note the 200-year-old tulip poplar tree hulking by the trail.

Carefully cross Reservoir Road at 44th Street, and follow the trail through the woodlands. On your left is the western edge of Georgetown University, and on the right is the tony neighborhood of Foxhall. Here is where you come to a deteriorating trestle bridge that was used by the trolley to Glen Echo amusement park. If you encounter a detour sign and fence prohibiting hikers and bikers, turn back for safety's sake.

If there are no detour signs, follow the dirt trail until you come to Foxhall and Canal Roads. On the other side of the roads is the C&O Canal Towpath. Without crossing these busy roads, you'll have a view of Rosslyn's high-rises in the distance. Retrace your steps to return to the trailhead.

NEARBY/RELATED ACTIVITIES

Explore downtown Georgetown and its many restaurants and shops. During the warmer months, rent a kayak at Fletcher's Boathouse (202-337-9642, boatingindc .com). In American University Park, visit the Katzen Arts Center (202-885-2787, american.edu/cas/katzen) on the American University campus. Tour the Washington National Cathedral (202-537-6200, cathedral.org) just a few blocks from here.

· ·

GPS TRAILHEAD COORDINATES N38° 56.046' W77° 04.854'

DIRECTIONS From I-495, take Exit 39 to merge onto River Road East toward Washington, D.C. Turn right onto Ridgefield Road. Then turn left onto Westbard Avenue. Turn left onto Massachusetts Avenue and drive around Westmoreland Circle, entering the District of Columbia. Continue on Massachusetts Avenue past American University, and park near Macomb Street and the Washington Hebrew Congregation. For public transportation, take the Metro to Tenleytown–AU Station. Take the N2 bus to American University Park. Contact Metro, 202-637-7000 or wmata.com.

6 KENILWORTH AQUATIC GARDENS AND THE ANACOSTIA RIVERWALK TRAIL

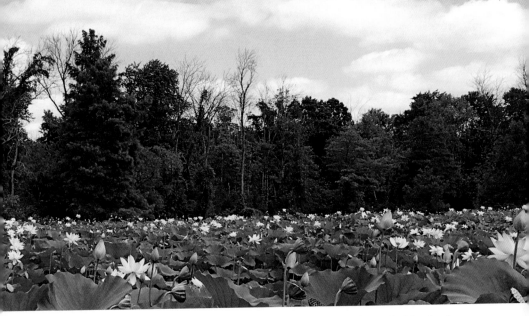

Kenilworth Aquatic Gardens is home to both cultivated, historic water gardens and wild wetlands.

THE KENILWORTH AQUATIC GARDENS and Kenilworth Marsh constitute an alluring botanical gem and a hiking locale worth visiting in any season. The new connection to the Anacostia Riverwalk Trail allows the option to extend the length of the hike beyond the national park.

DESCRIPTION

For a short and exotic urban hike that's wonderfully nonurban, visit the Kenilworth Aquatic Gardens and adjoining 77-acre Kenilworth Marsh, located on the east bank of the Anacostia River. There you'll find a combination of garden landscape and mini-wilderness in the collective form of gorgeous water-lily ponds (also a summer-time butterfly hot spot), wildflower-infused woodlands, a plant- and wildlife-rich tidal marsh, and a lovely air of serenity. This trail incorporates the entire boundary of the national park and includes 2 miles on the new Anacostia Riverwalk Trail. The first leg is on a woodland trail that travels through Kenilworth Gardens to access the Riverwalk Trail. The second is a stroll down and back on the paved Riverwalk Trail. The third section explores the 12-acre lily-pond area.

LENGTH 4.9 miles (with shorter options)

CONFIGURATION Out-and-back with a loop

DIFFICULTY Very easy

SCENERY Water-lily ponds, marshlands, woodlands, boardwalk, Anacostia River, recreational activities

EXPOSURE Mostly exposed; some shade in the park, but no shade on the Anacostia Riverwalk

TRAFFIC Light–medium; heavy during the Lotus and Water Lily Festival

TRAIL SURFACE Mostly hard-packed, pebbly dirt; gravel, grass, boardwalk, pavement

HIKING TIME 2–2.5 hours (allowing for bird- and butterfly-watching)

DRIVING DISTANCE 6 miles

SEASON Year-round

ACCESS Open daily, 8 a.m.–4 p.m., November 1–March 31; open daily, 9 a.m. –5 p.m., April 1–October 31 (closed Thanksgiving Day, Christmas Day, and New Year's Day)

WHEELCHAIR TRAVERSABLE On the Anacostia Riverwalk

MAPS USGS *Washington East*; sketch map in free gardens pamphlet

FACILITIES Restrooms, water, and phones at visitor center; water and restrooms at Kenilworth Parkside Recreational Park

CONTACT 202-692-6080, nps.gov/keaq

LOCATION Southeast Washington, D.C.

COMMENTS Be sure to leave the park by 4 or 5 p.m., when the outer entrance gate is closed; additional access from Anacostia Riverwalk during hours of operation. No charge to enter.

In planning a Kenilworth visit, remember that the water-lily blooming season lasts from May until September, with color lingering into early November. The hardy lilies, which stay outside year-round, have blooms that open during the day and are at their peak in June and July. The lotuses and other tropical lilies, which winter in greenhouses, are at their flowering best in July and August. They include both day bloomers and night bloomers. On a morning visit, you'll see—and smell—the day bloomers as they open and the night bloomers before they close. Remember, too, that the park can be glorious any time of year. Winter, for instance, is a lovely time to hike around the marsh and on the less busy Riverwalk Trail.

To get started from the visitor parking lot, head toward the visitor center, which has restrooms, a bookstore, and maps. You can also check to see when the rangers are leading groups through the marshes. Leave the visitor center, and turn right toward the signposted Marsh & River Trail.

The dirt trail winds through deciduous woods for three-quarters of a mile, and you'll catch glimpses of the marsh and waterfowl, and perhaps a muskrat or otter. The trail ends by linking the Anacostia Riverwalk Trail to the marsh, then heads either north or south. Turn left (away from the train bridge) at the signpost, and begin hiking on the Riverwalk Trail, being careful to avoid fast-moving cyclists.

The Riverwalk Trail is a 20-mile multiuse trail with a combination of boardwalks and pavement. The trail was designed to link the east and west banks of the Anacostia River stretching from the new Wharf development to Prince George's

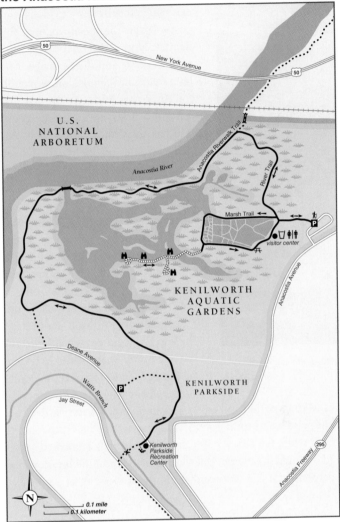

Kenilworth Aquatic Gardens and the Anacostia Riverwalk Trail

County, Maryland. Twelve miles of trail were completed in late 2016, including this stretch. Eventually, the trail will allow pedestrians and bicyclists to walk from the Fish Market and Nationals Park, past the National Arboretum, and ultimately end up at Bladensburg Marina Park in Maryland.

Stay on the Riverwalk Trail, passing the Kenilworth Landfill and parking area and then ending at the Kenilworth Parkside Recreation Center near the Eastland

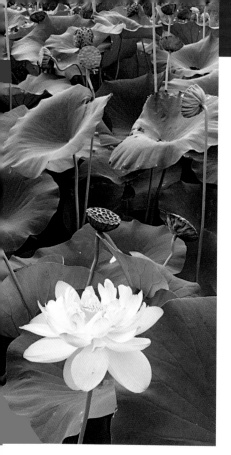

The lilies and lotuses are at their peak blooming period in June and July.

Gardens neighborhood. During this walk, you can take a few detours to check out the Anacostia River, the meadows, and the wetlands habitat. Notice the tidal pools where wildlife such as geese and ducks thrive. After the athletic fields and tennis courts, you'll see a sign for Anacostia Park. At the playground, turn around to walk back the way you came until you reenter Kenilworth Gardens. Make a right and walk back on the Marsh & River Trail.

Turn right at the sign for the boardwalk, and head out over the wetlands. The boardwalks pass over the acres of lilies and other water plants. Along this walk, be sure to stop at the three observation areas. After that, walk back toward the visitor center. There's a nice place for a picnic, or you can return to the parking lot. If you prefer a 2-mile hike, eliminate the Anacostia Riverwalk section.

Kenilworth Aquatic Gardens dates back to the late 19th century, when a government clerk named Walter Shaw planted a dozen lilies from his native Maine in an old farm pond. His hobby soon became a business. New ponds were dug, exotic species were imported and cultivated, and Shaw's water gardens became both a thriving enterprise and a tourist attraction. In the late 1930s, though, the gardens seemed doomed when the U.S. Army Corps of Engineers embarked on dredging the Anacostia and draining the marsh. But the Department of the Interior stepped in and bought the gardens—for $15,000—and made them the core of a new National Park Service unit.

Information boards introduce visitors to the ecology of a freshwater tidal marsh. You'll see such native plants as cattails, sedges, American lotus, and wild rice and much sky. Where the boardwalk ends, it's possible to see herons and egrets fishing, ducks bobbing, or an osprey or bald eagle flapping by. Look out for beavers that slip into the ponds, mostly at night, to feast on water lily roots. Contemplate, or even marvel at, the existence of such a place within the city limits.

The marshlands are a remnant of the area's original wetlands. In the summer and early fall, on view are the spectacular South American tropical lilies called *Victoria amazonica,* with their huge floating pads and night-blooming, football-size flowers. The rangers are usually out and about, so stop to ask them about the various water plants, such as the exotic East Indian lotus descended from centuries-old seeds discovered in Manchuria in 1951.

NEARBY/RELATED ACTIVITIES

There's much to do at Kenilworth. Tour the exhibit-packed visitor center. Talk to the rangers. Take a ranger-guided morning tour of the ponds (call for details). Arrange to take a canoe trip through the marshes with the Anacostia Watershed Society, 301-699-6204 or anacostiaws.org. Just across the Anacostia River is the United States National Arboretum (Hike 11, page 62). The two locales complement one another: Kenilworth provides exotic aquatic gardens and an all-American marsh with its avian residents and visitors, while the arboretum offers a rich sampling of plants from several continents. Both locales have views found nowhere else in the city.

• •

GPS TRAILHEAD COORDINATES N38° 54.794' W76° 56.414'

DIRECTIONS From downtown Washington, take New York Avenue Northeast (US 50) heading out of town (northeast). After passing the Bladensburg Road intersection and the United States National Arboretum, go about 2 miles and turn right onto Kenilworth Avenue (MD 201). Head south 0.4 mile toward I-295, and then take the first right (watch for the sign for Addison Road and Eastern Avenue) onto Kenilworth Avenue frontage road. Follow the large brown AQUATIC GARDENS signs. Go straight at the Eastern Avenue junction, proceed two blocks, and turn right onto Douglas Street. Go 0.3 mile to the end of Douglas, and turn right onto Anacostia Avenue. Then turn left through the gate into the visitor parking lot—the trailhead. *Note:* Leaving the gardens can be tricky because of one-way streets; one option is to return to Douglas Street and the Kenilworth Avenue frontage road; turn right onto the one-way frontage road; go 1.5 miles; turn right onto Benning Road; go right onto 17th Street; and then, at Bladensburg Road, go either right toward New York Avenue or left toward the Capitol Hill area.

7 ROCK CREEK PARK:
Boulder Bridge Trail

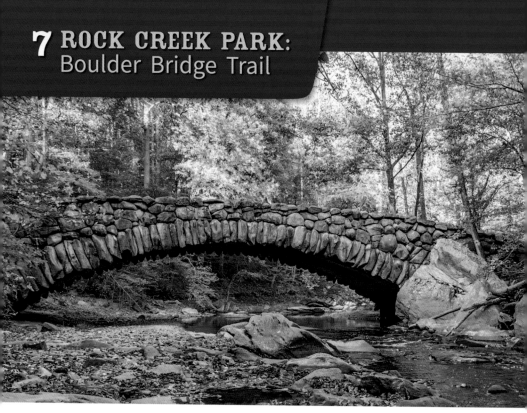

Historic Boulder Bridge crossing Rock Creek is this hike's namesake.

NORTHERN ROCK CREEK PARK is a haven of wilderness inside the city boundaries. There are historic sites and multiple trails inside the park. The National Park Service manages Rock Creek Park; the hiking, biking, and horseback riding trails; and all the concessions. There are multiple places to picnic and enjoy nature along the trail.

DESCRIPTION

To begin your hike on the Boulder Bridge Trail, park at the Rock Creek Park Nature Center and Planetarium. The facilities are accessed from Military Road, just north of the National Zoo. The nature center has restrooms and a small bookstore with merchandise pertaining to the region. The ranger can provide a trail map with descriptions of several hikes.

Start out walking past the horse barn and corral, until you see a trailhead at the end of the small parking lot. Look for the pink blaze on a wooden pole, and keep your eyes peeled for those pink blazes throughout the hike. After the trailhead, the trail descends slightly as you walk through the forest. You'll pass an enormous fallen tree that has been cut in half to allow for the trail to pass through. Look out for the occasional horse manure in the middle of the trail. The forest consists of saplings

LENGTH 3.7 miles (with longer options)

CONFIGURATION Loop

DIFFICULTY Moderate, with some difficult parts

SCENERY Rolling woodlands, creek valley, boulder bridges, horse stables

EXPOSURE Mostly shady; less so in winter

TRAFFIC Usually very light–light

TRAIL SURFACE Mostly dirt or stony dirt; some pavement; rocky and rooty in places

HIKING TIME 3–4 hours (including visit to nature center and horse center)

DRIVING DISTANCE 7 miles

SEASON Year-round

ACCESS Open daily, sunrise–sunset

WHEELCHAIR TRAVERSABLE No

MAPS Sketch map in free NPS Rock Creek Park brochure; tinyurl.com/rockcreekmap

FACILITIES Horse barn and stables; restrooms, water, and gift shop at nature center; planetarium

CONTACT 202-895-6000 or nps.gov/rocr

LOCATION Washington, D.C.

COMMENTS These trails are not well marked and can be confusing to follow. Be sure take a trail map with you. Don't hesitate to use GPS or a compass to help you stay on course. Because it can be difficult to find your footing on the rocky and rooty spots, avoid hiking this trail after a heavy rain.

and some old-growth hardwoods. All are deciduous—mostly oak, beech, maple, and tulip trees—so it's shady in the warmer months. The path is wide enough for two here and is well maintained.

Make a slight left and walk down the hill toward Ross Drive where it intersects Military Road. At the bottom of the hill, there's a picnic table and an information sign about Rock Creek Park. Here's where you begin walking along a path that parallels Rock Creek. As you follow the path, you'll enjoy the sound of rapids and the view of the roaring creek as it cuts through impressive rock formations. This geologic transition zone is where the harder rock of the Piedmont Plateau meets the softer sedimentary rock of the Atlantic Coastal Plain.

You'll pass a little stone house and more picnic benches, and the first bridge you come to is Rapids Bridge. Look up the hill to your right as you hike along the creek; you'll pass a giant boulder with a huge tree trunk growing out of it. You'll encounter multiple elevations on this hilly riverbank, with views of the water and gigantic boulders that wrap around the river. Look left, across Beach Drive, to see the office of the U.S. Park Police housed in a historic building.

The next waypoint you'll encounter is Boulder Bridge, one of the oldest bridges in the park, constructed in 1902. First, cross over Boulder Bridge, and then carefully cross Beach Drive. On the east side of Beach Drive, you'll see a pink blaze designating the Valley Trail. You'll turn right here, following the pink blazes that point uphill. Watch your footing as you make your way along this rocky, uneven trail.

It's also a bit confusingly marked, thanks to a combination of both blue and pink blazes on the trees. Continue following the pink blazes for the Valley Trail. At the

Rock Creek Park: Boulder Bridge Trail

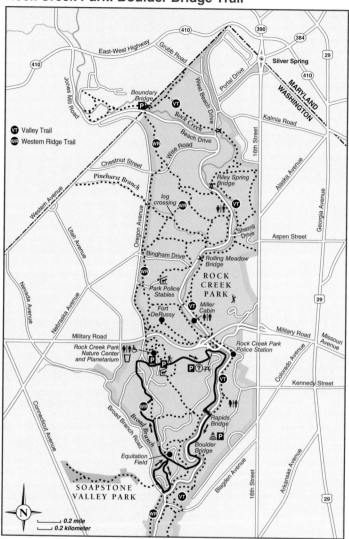

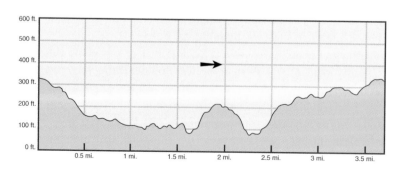

bottom of the hill you'll see a pink blaze marking the turn to the right on the trail, and cross back over Beach Drive to enter the Western Ridge Trail marked with green blazes. This is a scenic spot where you can get down close to the river and take in a beautiful view of the park. Before continuing on the trail, walk down to the sandy beach to see the ducks. The ground by the riverbank is very soft and offers a nice place to rest or picnic.

As you follow Western Ridge Trail's green blazes, you'll see Rock Creek below and pass by a barn to your left. Continue climbing up the hill on an uneven surface with a substantial elevation. At the top of the hill, stay straight at the four-way intersection. Continue toward the pink blaze across the street, and follow the pink blazes toward the Equitation Field, a pen for horse jumping. At this point, you have two choices: you can walk past the field straight ahead on the Western Ridge Trail back toward the Nature Center, or you can turn left to get some extra hiking in. For an additional mile, follow the green blazes to the left on the Oak-Beech/Heath Hike used by horses and hikers. This trail involves climbing up a very steep incline and then back down before returning to the Equitation Field.

If you stay on the Western Ridge Trail, you'll see a sign that says NO HORSES. The dirt trail now meanders through a forest marked with green blazes. A few paces after you cross a boardwalk, you'll carefully cross Grant Road and then Glover Road. Walk up the steps toward the nature center and picnic area 13. Keep heading uphill toward the parking lot to finish the hike.

There are multiple side trips and shortcuts as well. Rather than the full loop, you can cut across the park to the west at Rapids Bridge to head back to the Nature Center, or use one of the lateral trails shown on the map to cut across the basic loop.

NEARBY/RELATED ACTIVITIES

The National Zoo (202-633-4888, nationalzoo.si.edu) is located inside Rock Creek Park. Go for a trail ride at Rock Creek Park Horse Center (202-362-0117, rockcreek horsecenter.com), or play golf at the 18-hole public Rock Creek Park Golf Course (202-882 7332, golfdc.com/rock-creek-gc). Visit Hillwood Museum Estate and Gardens (202-686-5807, hillwoodmuseum.org), a mansion once owned by Marjorie Merriweather Post that has exquisite gardens, house tours, and regular events.

• •

GPS TRAILHEAD COORDINATES N38° 57.528' W77° 02.964'

DIRECTIONS Head for Northwest Washington. From the intersection of Connecticut and Nebraska Avenues, head northeast on Nebraska 0.4 mile. Make an easy (not sharp) right onto Military Road and drive east 0.7 mile. Then turn right, south, onto Glover Road to enter Rock Creek Park. Proceed

0.4 mile, swinging left at the fork and then taking the first left to get to the parking lot for Rock Creek Nature Center and Planetarium.

Or use the Metro and your feet: From either Friendship Heights Metro station (Red line) or Fort Totten Metro station (Red and Green lines), take Metrobus E2 or E3 along Military Road. Get off at Oregon Avenue (opposite Glover Road). From the southeast corner of the intersection, walk uphill on the paved path 0.2 mile to reach the trailhead. Contact Metro, 202-637-7000 or wmata.com.

Meet the park rangers and tour Rock Creek Park Nature Center. It has exhibits on area plants and animals, as well as a planetarium.

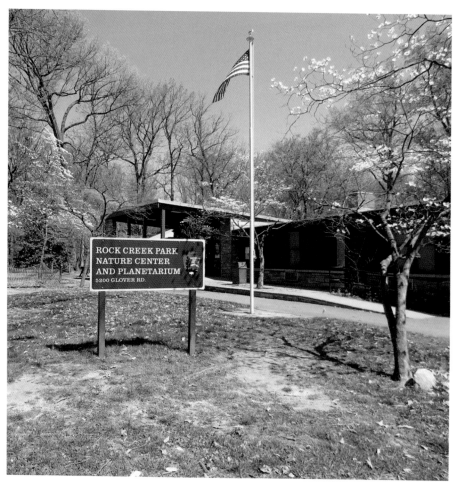

8 ROCK CREEK PARK:
Northern Section

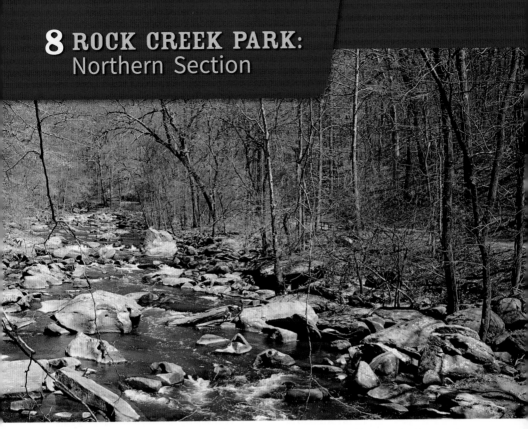

The hiking trails in Rock Creek Park extend from D.C. into Maryland and provide a great place to enjoy green space within the urban boundaries.

THE HILLY AND LITTLE-USED WOODLANDS of Rock Creek Park's northern section rank as one of Washington's best venues for off-street hiking in a wilderness-tinged setting.

DESCRIPTION

The same year that Congress granted national park status to the three big chunks of California known as Yosemite, Sequoia, and Kings Canyon, it also preserved a piece of its own backyard, decreeing that Rock Creek's valley would become "a pleasuring ground for the benefit and enjoyment of the people of the United States." That was in 1890. Today, covering about 2,100 acres, the park consists largely of woodlands and stream valleys that provide habitat for assorted flora and fauna. Most visitors head for the picnic areas or other recreation facilities, but informed hikers head for the hills and trails.

This 6.8-mile hike consists of a modified loop that accumulates about 700 feet of elevation change. The major trails are blazed, named, and signposted. There are lots of unmarked trails that take you out of the park, so be sure to follow the blazes. And there are several cross-park trails that you can use to create shorter hikes (see

LENGTH 6.8 miles (with longer and shorter options)

CONFIGURATION Loop

DIFFICULTY Moderate

SCENERY Rolling woodlands, stream valleys

EXPOSURE Mostly shady; less so in winter

TRAFFIC Usually very light–light; heavier on warm-weather evenings, weekends, and holidays

TRAIL SURFACE Mostly dirt or stony dirt; some pavement; rocky and rooty in places

HIKING TIME 3.5 hours

DRIVING DISTANCE 7 miles

SEASON Year-round

ACCESS Open daily, sunrise–sunset

WHEELCHAIR TRAVERSABLE No

MAPS tinyurl.com/rockcreekmap

FACILITIES Restrooms, water, and phone at nature center (open Wednesday–Sunday, 9 a.m.–5 p.m.); restrooms near Riley Spring Bridge (warm season only)

CONTACT 202-895-6000, nps.gov/rocr

LOCATION Washington, D.C.

COMMENTS The trails in Rock Creek Park can be confusing to follow at some points as they are not well marked and have many intersections. Generally, you should be able to follow the color-coded blazes. The major trails are visible on Google Maps, so use a smartphone to verify your location if necessary.

the map). Rain makes the unpaved trails muddy; horses make them even muddier. Beware occasional flooding and winter iciness, and stay out of the poison ivy.

To get started from the nature center's parking lot, pick up the nearby nature trail at the north end, at an EDGE OF THE WOODS sign. Turn right onto the paved Western Ridge Trail. At Military Road, carefully cross, and stay on the path as it goes uphill and into the woods. At the Fort DeRussy sign, turn right. Then take a slight left onto the dirt trail. Watch for small yellow posts along the way, and continue past the Civil War–era fort named after Union brigadier general Rene Edward DeRussy. During the Battle of Fort Stevens in July 1864, Fort DeRussy's 100-pound guns fired more than 100 rounds into enemy lines, proving integral in stopping the attack and defending the nation's capital. When the trail merges, keep right and continue straight toward the bridge. Follow the trail underneath the bridge (Military Road), and then turn left to cross the bridge at Joyce Road. Turn left again onto Rock Creek Trail, which runs alongside the creek and to the left of Beach Drive. Cross under the bridge (Military Road) again, and immediately cross Beach Drive to take the narrow entrance to the blue-blazed Valley Trail, the major north–south trail on the park's eastern side.

Half a mile north of Military Road, you will pass Miller Cabin, a 19th-century log cabin built by American poet and essayist Joaquin Miller. The historic property is a rare log cabin structure made of split logs and chinking with a fieldstone fireplace. It was painstakingly deconstructed from its original site in Northwest Washington and moved to Rock Creek Park in 1911.

Keep watching for blue blazes and signposts for Boundary Bridge, ignoring the intersections with cross-park trails. As the creek parallels the road to your left, it

Rock Creek Park: Northern Section

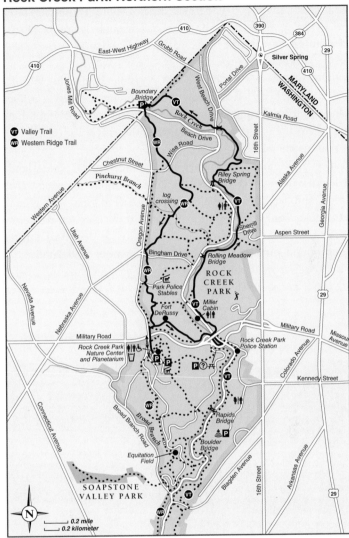

VT Valley Trail

WR Western Ridge Trail

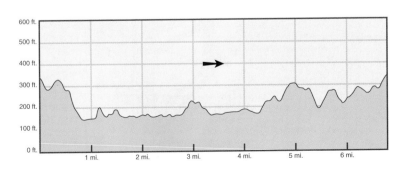

gives the impression of being a wilderness stream. Some sections are more secluded than others. In spring, this stretch of trail passes through one of the District's richest displays of wildflowers. So either soak up the color as you hike by, or slow down to savor whatever strikes your fancy.

Keep following the Valley Trail north, passing the Rolling Meadow Bridge. When the trail splits, keep left to follow the trail under the bridge at Sherrill Drive. After passing the Riley Spring Bridge, turn right and go steeply uphill onto a wide trail for a short stretch that strays away from the creek and nears the back of a residential neighborhood.

The Valley Trail ends at Boundary Bridge and the D.C.–Maryland border. A short paved path will take you to a small parking lot adjoining Beach Drive. Carefully cross the road, and head uphill on a narrow dirt trail marked with green blazes. It's the Western Ridge Trail, the major north–south trail along the western side of the park and your route back to the trailhead. You may see deer near this trail. On the 2.5-mile southbound journey, you'll pass through mature woodlands.

At Wise Road, cross wisely. Then press on, past a couple of cross-park trails. After that, you'll cross Pinehurst Branch, and the trail goes up a steep incline.

The park has miles of trails and many opportunities to linger by the creek.

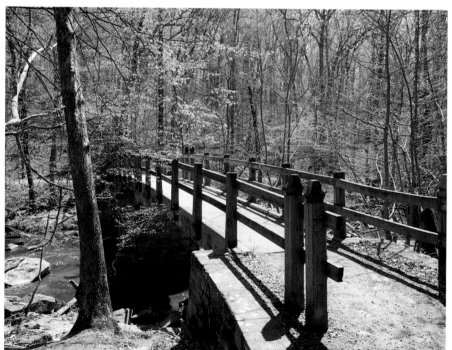

Stay on the Western Ridge Trail, crossing Bingham Drive. When you reach Horse Stable Road, there is a gap in the trail. Turn left and follow the gravel road a short distance until you see the dirt path emerge again on the right. Take a right back onto the Western Ridge Trail, and proceed into the woods, mostly downhill. Turn right at a junction (to the left is another cross-park trail), and continue, mostly upward. At the next junction, turn right (again, to the left is a cross-park trail). At Oregon Avenue the trail becomes paved once again. Follow the trail downhill toward Military Road, cross the street carefully, and then turn left and head for the Rock Creek Park Visitor Center.

NEARBY/RELATED ACTIVITIES

Visit the nature center and learn about the park's flora and fauna. Attend a park ranger program or tour the fully restored Peirce Mill (202-426-6908) and the nearby Rock Creek Gallery (long known as the Art Barn). After the hike, sample the Connecticut Avenue restaurants near the trailhead.

• •

GPS TRAILHEAD COORDINATES N38° 57.528' W77° 02.964'

DIRECTIONS Head for Northwest Washington. From the intersection of Connecticut and Nebraska Avenues, head northeast on Nebraska 0.4 mile. Make an easy (not sharp) right onto Military Road and drive east 0.7 mile. Then turn right, south, onto Glover Road to enter Rock Creek Park. Proceed 0.4 mile, swinging left at the fork and then taking the first left to get to the parking lot for Rock Creek Nature Center and Planetarium.

Or use the Metro and your feet: From either the Friendship Heights station (Red line) or Fort Totten Metro station (Red and Green lines), take Metrobus E2 or E3 along Military Road. Get off at Oregon Avenue (opposite Glover Road). From the southeast corner of the intersection, walk uphill on the paved path 0.2 mile to reach the trailhead. Contact Metro, 202-637-7000 or wmata.com.

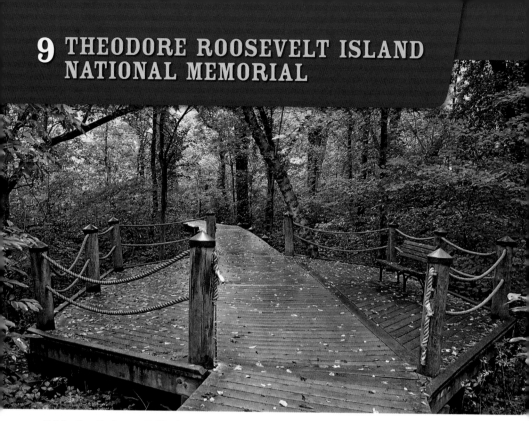

At 1.5 miles, the Swamp Trail is the island's longest. It passes through swampy woods and cattail marsh.

THIS CLOSE-IN POTOMAC RIVER ISLAND is a self-contained parkland with impressive views of Georgetown and Rosslyn. It features the Theodore Roosevelt Memorial and nature preserve, along with a picturesque boardwalk through wetlands and other trails.

DESCRIPTION

Metro-area hikers owe Theodore Roosevelt a grateful nod. During Roosevelt's 1901–09 presidency, the country got a forest service and wildlife-refuge system, and the metro area had a hiker in the White House. This 2.8-mile, hill-less hike, managed by the National Park Service, loops through the scenic parklands that surround the memorial. Trail signs are few, but the area is so small, you can't get lost for long.

The hike begins at the entryway to Theodore Roosevelt Island, which is surprisingly part of Washington, not Virginia. Long known as Analostan Island, it was a plantation until the Civil War and later a recreation area. Neglected for decades, it was bought by the Theodore Roosevelt Memorial Association in 1931 and given to the National Park Service. Taken on as a Civilian Conservation Corps project, the island was renamed, stripped of everything man-made, planted with 30,000 trees, and allowed to evolve as a nature preserve. The memorial was added in 1967.

LENGTH 2.8 miles (with shorter options)

CONFIGURATION Modified loop

DIFFICULTY Easy

SCENERY River and canal views, street scenes, parklands, woodlands

EXPOSURE Mostly open; more so in winter

TRAFFIC Light on weekdays; moderate–heavy on warm-weather evenings, weekends, and holidays

TRAIL SURFACE Pavement, dirt, boardwalk, brick

HIKING TIME 1.5–2 hours (depending on how often you stop to check out the views)

DRIVING DISTANCE 5 miles

SEASON Year-round

ACCESS Open daily, 6 a.m.–10 p.m.; no fees required; no bicycles allowed

WHEELCHAIR TRAVERSABLE Yes, on parts of the Swamp Trail and around the memorial

MAPS USGS *Washington West*; ADC *Metro Washington* and *Northern Virginia*; sketch map in free brochure and on bulletin board

FACILITIES Restrooms and water fountain open during summer months only

CONTACT George Washington Memorial Parkway Headquarters, 703-289-2500, nps.gov

LOCATION Arlington, Virginia

COMMENTS The island is very popular with local runners. Cars parked on the grass will be ticketed.

To get started, take the footbridge to the heavily wooded island, which is a great place for studying birds, trees, and wildflowers. As you cross the bridge, look north and you'll be able to see the spires of the National Cathedral and Georgetown University. Behind, you'll see the tall buildings of Rosslyn, and to the south you'll see Memorial Bridge.

There's a sign directing kids to follow a trail with a series of self-guided adventures. Another sign shows trails on the island—there's the Upland Trail in the center of the island; the Woods Trail, which is right after the Memorial Plaza; and the Swamp Trail, which is the longest and hugs the perimeter of the island, consisting mostly of a boardwalk over wetlands.

When you enter the island, make a quick right and then a quick left, so you can see the Roosevelt Memorial, boasting a statue, large fountains, and four concrete pillars with quotes by Roosevelt. The concrete plaza also has picnic tables and benches. If you have time, stop to read the four quotes showcasing the important aspects of Roosevelt's life: Youth, Manhood, The State, and Nature. The one that belongs in this book is his Nature quote:

> There is light in the hearty life of the open. There are no words that can tell the hidden spirit of the wilderness, that can reveal its mystery, its melancholy, and its charm. The nation behaves well if it treats the natural resources as assets, which must turn over to the next generation increased and not impaired in value. Conservation means development as much as it does protection.

Theodore Roosevelt Island National Memorial

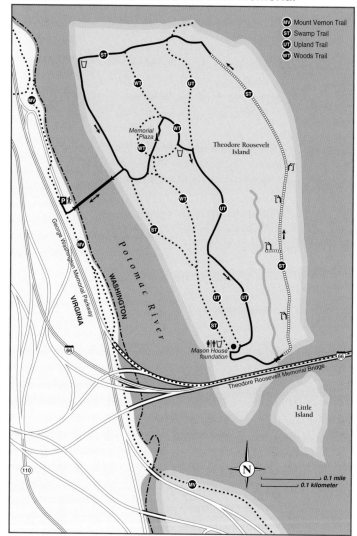

When you're ready to hike, walk behind the Roosevelt statue and look for the Woods Trail to the right. Take it for about 15 feet, until it dead-ends, and then turn right and continue 12 feet to the next intersection. Turn right to follow the Upland Trail to higher ground and through the woods, with an occasional view of the shoreline and river. This trail gets pretty muddy. You can't help but notice the constant sound of airplanes flying overhead on their way to Reagan National Airport just a few miles south.

The Upland Trail passes behind the memorial and by a water fountain. Keep walking straight, and look for the blue blazes. Occasionally, you might want to diverge to one of the many paths that lead to the shoreline so you can get a look at Washington Harbour across the river. You'll also see Key Bridge.

The forest is thick with hanging vines and the smell of sassafras. This is the natural habitat for many birds, including the ruby-throated hummingbird, white-breasted hatch, cardinal, catbird, mockingbird, Carolina wren, tufted titmouse, and downy woodpecker. Check out the sign with pictures of these birds to help you identify them. Other birds you might see are the mallard, barred owl, and great blue heron.

When you reach the loop intersection, take the left fork and walk until you come upon the sign that marks the site of the Mason House, circa 1818. There's a rendering of a map drawn by Robert King that portrays this island as one continuous garden, rich in native and cultivated plants, flowers, and fruit trees. Soon you'll see restrooms on the right, and the Swamp Trail heading to your left. Walk down the hill, and begin following the Swamp Trail, which is full of surprises.

First, you'll hear the loud noise of cars on the Roosevelt Memorial Bridge, also known as I-66. There's a fence intended to keep people off the bridge. When you walk underneath, look in the distance, and you can see the top of the Lincoln Memorial. Then turn left to cross a small wooden bridge over the swamp. Here is where the island lives up to its billing as a nature preserve. You'll begin hiking on a long boardwalk over lush, thriving marshlands, where you'll probably see ducks swimming through the cattails. The tide ebbs and flows here, and a sign mentions the marsh is an ideal habitat for crayfish (and for raccoons that love to eat them). Walk out onto the observation deck to get a panoramic view of the length of this epic swamp.

At the end of the boardwalk (you won't want it to end), you'll join a dirt trail and pass by a huge black boulder. Turn left and head back toward the parking lot. As you continue on the Swamp Trail toward the entrance, passing by the Causeway, you'll catch an imposing view of the high-rises that make up Rosslyn, Virginia. Return to the parking-lot trailhead, having hiked a meandering 2.8 miles.

NEARBY/RELATED ACTIVITIES

Arlington Cemetery (arlingtoncemetery.mil) is within walking distance of the island, and it's a beautiful place to walk and enjoy panoramic views of the National Mall, including the monuments and Tidal Basin. Stop at the Arlington House (703-235-1530, nps.gov/arho) for a tour of Robert E. Lee's former home and the slave quarters behind the house. The house has been refurbished to reflect the time before the Civil War, but the tour helps explain how the house functioned as a hospital and then a graveyard for Union soldiers. In nearby Rosslyn, visit the famous United States Marine Corps War Memorial (703-289-2500, nps.gov/gwmp), with its iconic statue of soldiers raising the flag after the Battle of Iwo Jima. Just a few miles away, visit the Pentagon Memorial (301-740-3388, pentagonmemorial.org), a serene place to honor those who lost their lives at the Pentagon on September 11, 2001.

• •

GPS TRAILHEAD COORDINATES N38° 53.754' W77° 04.001'

DIRECTIONS You can reach Theodore Roosevelt Island only from the northbound lanes of the George Washington Memorial Parkway. After Memorial Bridge, follow the sign to turn right into the parking lot. Or take the Metro to Rosslyn station and walk to the parking lot: From the station's main entrance, turn left and walk north (downhill) on North Moore Street, cross North 19th Street, turn right alongside Lee Highway, cross North Lynn Street, turn left and walk north on North Lynn, and cross Lee Highway. At the far corner, turn right onto the signposted Mount Vernon Trail, and follow it downhill, across the parkway and into the parking lot. Contact Metro, 202-637-7000 or wmata.com. By bicycle, take the Mount Vernon Trail. No bikes are allowed on the island.

Stop to read the speeches at the memorial describing President Roosevelt's commitment to preserving America's natural landscapes.

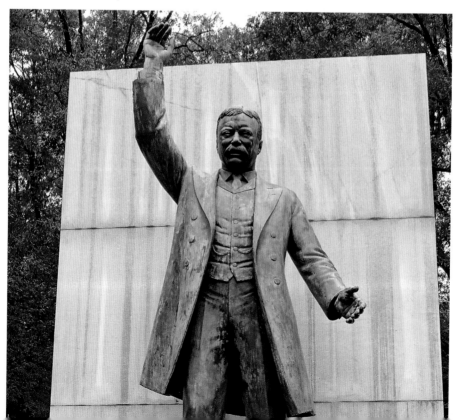

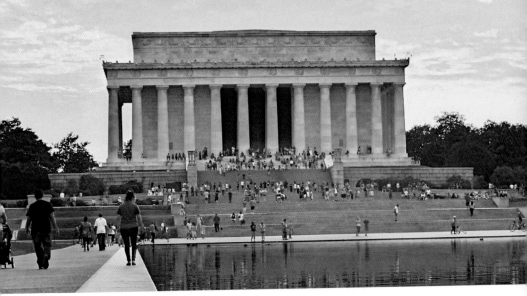

The Lincoln Memorial is one of the most iconic historic landmarks in Washington, D.C., and offers panoramic views of the National Mall.

ROAMING THE TIDAL BASIN and West Potomac Park on foot serves as a wonderful introduction to hiking in the nation's capital and to learning first-hand about the city's heritage and treasures.

DESCRIPTION

West Potomac Park is adjacent to the National Mall and the site of some of the most popular attractions in the nation's capital. The National Park Service refers to the Mall as "America's Front Yard—a public space that evokes the pride and patriotism of our nation." Visitors frequent the Mall's museums, monuments, and memorials and gather to play, picnic, stroll, jog, bike, relax, protest, march, and sightsee. The Mall, in effect, serves as the nation's town square, commons, pulpit, soapbox, park, and memorial garden. It's a great hiking venue where one can take self-propelled voyages of discovery and rediscovery, and it's small enough to cover on foot but large enough for a hiker to get some exercise—and avoid the crowds.

Note that "the Mall" usually refers to the grand 2.2-mile stretch of open space between the Lincoln Memorial and the U.S. Capitol. Officially, though, the Mall is only the part east of 14th Street, and the memorials themselves lie in West Potomac

LENGTH 4 miles (with shorter or longer options)

CONFIGURATION Loop

DIFFICULTY Easy–moderate

SCENERY Parklands, public buildings

EXPOSURE Mostly open

TRAFFIC Light–moderate; heavier in tourist season and on weekends and holidays

TRAIL SURFACE Mostly pavement

HIKING TIME 2 hours (plus additional time to visit the memorials)

DRIVING DISTANCE 1 mile

SEASON Year-round

ACCESS No restrictions

WHEELCHAIR TRAVERSABLE Partially accessible close to some of the memorials

MAPS USGS *Washington West*; ADC *Metro Washington*; posted map on display boards on and near West Potomac Park

FACILITIES Restrooms, water, and phones in museums and other public buildings on or near Mall; public restrooms on both sides of the Lincoln Memorial Reflecting Pool

CONTACT National Capital Parks, 202-619-7222, nps.gov/nacc

LOCATION Washington, D.C.

COMMENTS The National Mall is a high-security area. Obey signs, don't trespass, be prepared to modify your route if necessary, and finish hiking by dusk.

Park. The entire area is under National Park Service jurisdiction. While the area between the Smithsonian museums is open green space, this walk focuses on the Tidal Basin and West Potomac Park as the area is more parklike, encompassing a greater variety of trees, shrubs, and water features.

This 4-mile, clockwise loop begins at the Smithsonian Metro stop, circles around the Tidal Basin, extends to the Lincoln Memorial, and returns to the Metro station. It features sites of historical and cultural interest, with emphasis on presidents and, inevitably, war. It is planned as a daytime and outdoor hike, but you can detour indoors if you want; just maintain a good pace between stops, be careful crossing streets, and use the paths and sidewalks. For a shorter hike, you can consult a street map.

From the Smithsonian Metro station on the Mall, head south (toward Independence Avenue) about 20 yards. Turn right onto a broad paved path alongside Jefferson Drive. Follow the path across 14th and 15th Streets Northwest, and enjoy the view of the Washington Monument to your right. Turn left on 15th Street. Cross Independence Avenue and keep straight. You will pass the Holocaust Memorial Museum and the Bureau of Engraving and Printing on the left and see signs for East Potomac and West Potomac Parks. When you reach Maine Avenue, cross carefully and stay on the crosswalk. The Tidal Basin is straight ahead. As you pass by the basin boat rentals, stop to marvel at the view of the dome-shaped Jefferson Memorial. Follow the paved trail along the water to the left. Walk over a bridge and turn right to stay close to the water and walk toward the Jefferson Memorial. As you reach the memorial, step inside to view the 19-foot bronze statue and some of the inspiring

Tidal Basin and West Potomac Park

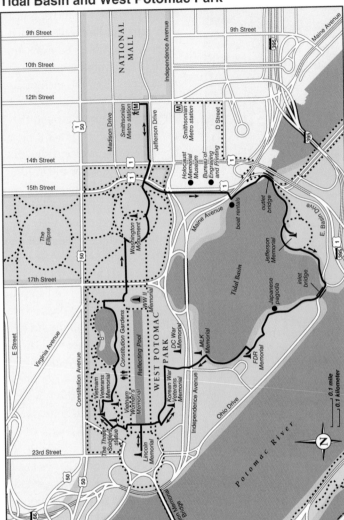

words of our third president. From the steps, enjoy panoramic views that include Rosslyn, Virginia; the Washington Monument; and even a peek at the White House.

After viewing the memorial, continue along the water until you come to a stop sign. Make a right to cross the bridge and follow the trail toward the Franklin Delano Roosevelt (FDR) Memorial. Pass the Japanese Stone Lantern on your right, and

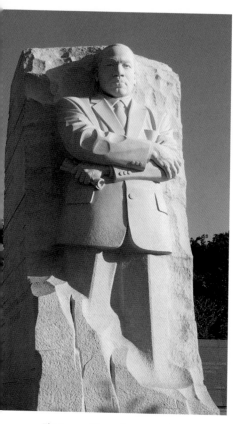

The Stone of Hope, the statue of Martin Luther King Jr., was designed by Chinese sculptor Lei Yixin.

continue to the memorial. It is a unique site with four outdoor galleries that are handicapped accessible. Be sure to check out some of the sculptures and read some of the inscriptions. Exit the memorial, go down a set of steps toward the water, and proceed left as you continue around the Tidal Basin toward the Martin Luther King Jr. Memorial. The memorial, dedicated in 2011, features a 30-foot granite statue of Dr. King and a 450-foot wall, made from granite panels, that is inscribed with 14 excerpts of King's sermons and public addresses. View the memorial, and then exit from the main entrance onto Independence Avenue (straying away from the Tidal Basin).

Cross the street, and continue across a dirt path that leads to the Lincoln Memorial Reflecting Pool. Walking straight ahead, on the right you will see the DC War Memorial, a circular bandstand, built in 1931 as Washington's World War I memorial. Turn left to walk toward the Lincoln Memorial. There, turn left and tour the Korean War Veterans Memorial. Dedicated in 1995, it depicts soldiers in winter. Made of stainless steel, the grim figures are reflected in a polished black granite wall on which many faces are faintly etched. Return to the intersection, head for the nearby Lincoln Memorial, and climb the 56 steps (Lincoln died at age 56). Enter the great chamber to face the seated marble figure that's four-and-a-half times life-size. Notice Lincoln's fingers, bent to form the letters *A* and *L* in sign language (Lincoln supported education for the deaf, and sculptor Daniel French had a deaf son). An inscription above Lincoln's head celebrates his having saved the Union but ignores his role in ending slavery. As the writer later explained, the memorial—opened in 1922—was meant to help heal the North–South rift, so it was best to "avoid the rubbing of old sores." But architect Henry Bacon had the chamber walls inscribed with the Gettysburg Address and the second inaugural address, which make clear Lincoln's views. Before leaving, look for the inscription marking the spot where Martin Luther King Jr. delivered his "I Have a Dream" speech in 1963.

Descend the steps, swing left, and head for the Vietnam Veterans Memorial. After passing an information kiosk, stop near a flagpole to see *The Three Soldiers* sculpture. Then take the paved path along the base of a sunken black granite wall carrying the names of the Vietnam War dead and missing. When dedicated in 1982, the memorial, designed by Maya Lin, consisted solely of the engraved wall. As she later wrote, "I did not want to civilize war by glorifying it or by forgetting the sacrifices involved." But her design provoked controversy, which led to *The Three Soldiers* being added in 1984. The nearby Vietnam Women's Memorial, showing three nurses aiding a fallen soldier, was added in 1993.

From there, retrace your steps to the last junction, and walk straight (east) on a paved path through Constitution Gardens. At a small lake, stay right and follow the paved waterside path to an elevated plaza. From there, follow the trail right to view the oval-shaped World War II Memorial, opened in 2004, combining granite, bronze, and fountains to create a peaceful place to remember those who served our country during that war.

Cross 17th Street and proceed to the first paved path leading to the sublimely abstract Washington Monument. When finished in 1884, the shaft topped out at about 555.5 feet. It's still the city's tallest masonry structure. Pass Sylvan Theater, the monument's outdoor stage, and keep straight to cross 15th and 14th Streets to return to the Smithsonian Metro station.

NEARBY/RELATED ACTIVITIES

During or after the hike, explore the nearby museums, including The National Museum of American History (202-633-1000, americanhistory.si.edu) and The National Museum of Natural History (202-633-1000, naturalhistory.si.edu). If you're hungry, stop by the Ronald Reagan Building and International Trade Center's food court on the lower level (202-312-1300, itcdc.com). The Federal Triangle Metro Station is across the courtyard.

• •

GPS TRAILHEAD COORDINATES N38° 53.343' W77° 01.690'

> **DIRECTIONS** Park near the trailhead at the Smithsonian Metro station entrance within the Mall (near Independence Avenue and 12th Street). Arrive early on crowded warm-weather weekends and holidays; heed local parking regulations. Or use the Metro: Smithsonian station is on the Orange and Blue lines; Metrobuses operate on nearby streets. Contact Metro, 202-637-7000 or wmata.com.

11 UNITED STATES NATIONAL ARBORETUM

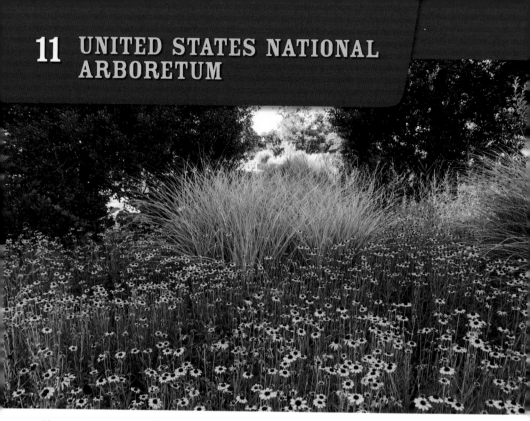

The National Arboretum offers endless opportunities to enjoy beautiful flowers, plants, and trees.

TUCKED AWAY IN NORTHEASTERN WASHINGTON, the United States National Arboretum ranks among the city's finest outdoor treasures and is this book's most botanically diverse hiking venue.

DESCRIPTION

Wedged between New York Avenue and the Anacostia River, the 446-acre arboretum serves primarily as a United States Department of Agriculture horticultural research center of global renown. However, for those of us who know, it's also a spacious and exotic recreational area that can dazzle the senses, intrigue the mind, restore the spirit, and exercise the body. Visitors can explore the mostly paved site on foot, by bike, and by car. There is also a 48-passenger open-air tram that offers a 35-minute public tour for a fee of $4 per adult and $2 for children ages 4–16 (free for children under 4). Tram rides run at noon, 1, 2, and 3 p.m. on weekends and holidays only.

Although the gently rolling woodlands and grassy open spaces seem serenely naturalistic, the landscape is thoroughly man-made. It represents the transformation of a tract of traditional American farmland into a thriving, one-of-a-kind botanical community consisting of many kinds of plants from around the world. The scenery

LENGTH 5.3 miles (with shorter options)

CONFIGURATION Modified loop

DIFFICULTY Moderate

SCENERY Woodlands, open spaces, exotic plants, odd structures

EXPOSURE Mostly open

TRAFFIC Generally very light–light; much heavier on spring weekends

TRAIL SURFACE Mostly paved; some dirt, gravel, concrete, grass, mulch

HIKING TIME 2.5–3 hours (plus time for lingering to take in the sights)

DRIVING DISTANCE 3 miles

ACCESS Open daily, 8 a.m.–5 p.m. (closed on December 25)

WHEELCHAIR TRAVERSABLE Yes, except the Asian Collections and the Capitol Columns

MAPS USGS *Washington East*; sketch map in free arboretum brochure

FACILITIES Restroom and water at administration building; restrooms at Arbor House and (warm-weather months only) near National Grove of State Trees and in Asian Collections

CONTACT 202-245-2726, usna.usda.gov

LOCATION Washington, D.C.

COMMENTS The visitor center is open 8 a.m.–4:30 p.m., the National Bonsai & Penjing Museum closes at 4 p.m., gates leading to the riverbank close at 4:30 p.m., and the arboretum's entrance gates clang shut at 5 p.m. Note that the street names are not thoroughly marked and the maps provided by the arboretum are not very detailed. The best way to navigate the site is using Google Maps from a smartphone. The site is well mapped out using an online GPS.

changes with each passing season, and with plants blooming in all 12 months, the arboretum is an educationally and aesthetically rewarding venue at any time of year.

Starting at the visitor center, make a left out the front door and then a right onto Meadow Road. Turn right onto Hickey Lane in front of the Friendship Garden, walking past the R Street entrance and parking lot. The walk here is on paved road with full sun exposure. Pass the first intersection and keep straight on Hickey Lane. Admire the bordering maples as the road begins to gradually slope uphill. At the next intersection, take a left again to stay on Hickey Lane, and then turn right onto Conifer Road. Watch on your right for the Gotelli collection, a 5-acre Lilliputian forest of dwarf conifers donated by ardent collector William Gotelli in 1962 and worth a detour. Let yourself be amazed by the single-trunk weeping blue Atlas cedar and other beauties. Also meander through a lovely azalea grove.

To view the Asian Collections, take a left and walk down a stone path to the Japanese Woodland. The path becomes gravel and enters the Asian Valley. Take a right into the China Valley, which becomes a paved trail and slopes downhill. You will come to a gate and a picnic area that overlooks the Anacostia River. After enjoying the view, walk back up the hill to the next intersection and continue straight on Hickey Hill Road. Pause there to sample the arboretum's hollies and magnolias. Turn left onto Crabtree Road. Pass the Youth Garden with white-blossomed crape myrtle and you will see the Capitol Columns to the right. Keep straight, as you will get a closer view later in the hike. Pass the Grove of State Trees picnic area, and

United States National Arboretum

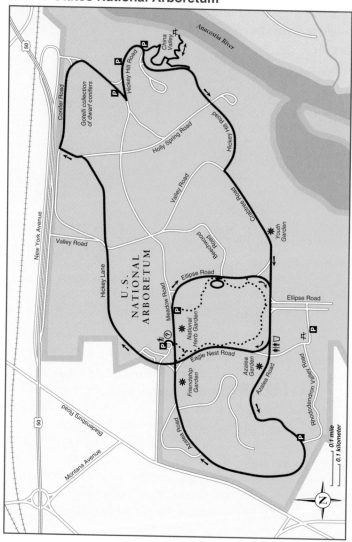

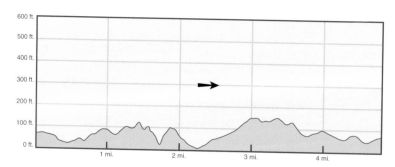

continue onto Azalea Road. Stop to view the Azalea Collection, and then continue along Azalea Road. As you proceed, you will see Mount Olivet Cemetery on the left and eventually the Washington Monument and the Basilica of the National Shrine. This road will return you to the visitor center.

From the visitor center, take the path to explore the exquisite National Bonsai & Penjing Museum (which closes at 4 p.m.). Also roam through the nearby National Herb Garden, where there's much to both smell and see, including old varieties of roses and 800 kinds of herbs. In summer, look for water lilies and flashy carp in the administration building's patio ponds. Continue south to see the National Capitol Columns, 22 capital-topped sandstone columns arranged in austere, Acropolis-like splendor on a low knoll. The columns were installed there in 1990, three decades after completing their first assignment—supporting the Capitol's east portico for 130 years—and after being stored, allegedly, in Kenilworth Marsh. Continue walking south on Ellipse Road, and you will come to the National Grove of State Trees, where trees representing each state have been planted. Make a right at Eagle Nest Road and continue back to the visitor center and parking lot.

NEARBY/RELATED ACTIVITIES

Visit the Arbor House gift shop (open March–mid-December, Monday–Friday, 10 a.m.–3 p.m., and Saturday–Sunday, 10 a.m.–5 p.m.). Combine this hike with Hike 6 (page 37). Contact the arboretum to learn about its volunteer opportunities and its many program offerings, especially the 5-mile full-moon hikes and plant sales.

• •

GPS TRAILHEAD COORDINATES N38° 54.750' W76° 58.217'

DIRECTIONS From downtown Washington, D.C., take New York Avenue Northeast (US 50) heading out of town. Turn right onto Bladensburg Road. Drive about 0.4 mile and turn left onto R Street, which ends in 0.2 mile at the arboretum's main entrance. Drive through the gates to the parking lot. Or, while on New York Avenue, cross Bladensburg Road to swing right onto a service road leading to the other gated entrance; once inside, bear right and follow Hickey Lane to the R Street parking lot. Note: To access westbound New York Avenue after the hike, get back on R Street, turn right onto Bladensburg Road, and then take the first left, onto Montana Avenue, which runs into New York Avenue.

Or travel by Metro. Take the Orange or Blue line to Stadium Armory Metro station, transfer to Metrobus B2, leave the bus at Bladensburg Road and R Street, and walk 0.2 mile along R Street.

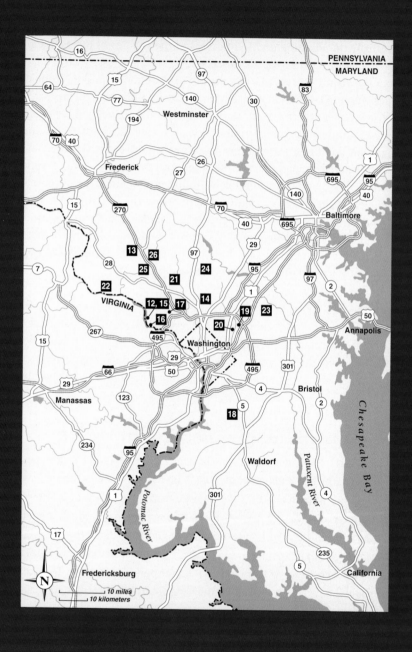

CLOSE-IN MARYLAND SUBURBS (Parts of Montgomery and Prince George's Counties)

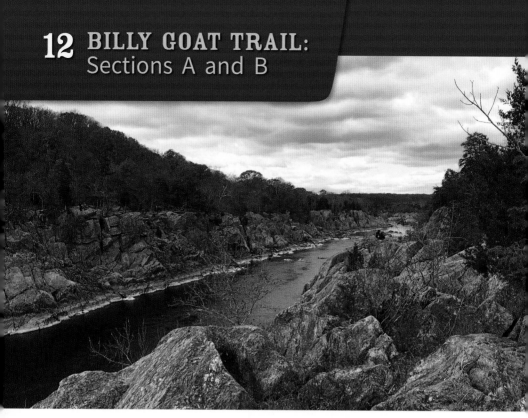

The trail features some of the best views of the Potomac and great photography opportunities.

OFFERING CLOSE-UP VIEWS of the thundering Great Falls as well as calmer sections of the Potomac River, the Billy Goat Trail is a favorite for local hikers. It has three segments: A (1.7 miles), B (1.4 miles), and C (1.6 miles). Each section connects to the C&O Canal Towpath and can be hiked independently with a return loop along the towpath. Part A is the most challenging and most popular. Parts B and C are mostly level and less crowded.

DESCRIPTION

This 8-mile hike includes about 2 miles of challenging rock scrambling and 6 miles of easier terrain. It begins on the C&O Canal Towpath near Great Falls Tavern, follows sections A and B along the river, and then returns on a level path combining the towpath with a 1.5-mile loop along Berma Road, an old conduit road that parallels the canal. The hike is challenging and offers a variety of views and terrain.

Great Falls Tavern, a historic landmark that dates from the late 1820s, long served as a lockhouse, hotel, or both. It's now a visitor center with museum exhibits. Begin your hike here and cross over the C&O Canal at lock 20; then turn left and proceed along the towpath for nearly a mile. Pass the pedestrian bridge to Great Falls Overlook at Olmsted Island just before lock 17, or take a short side trip to view

LENGTH 8 miles (with shorter or longer options)

CONFIGURATION Modified loop

DIFFICULTY Easy–difficult

SCENERY River and canal views, woodlands

EXPOSURE Open and wooded; less so in winter

TRAFFIC Section A is usually busy; section B is less busy; heavier on warm-weather evenings, weekends, and holidays

TRAIL SURFACE Hard-packed dirt on towpath and section B; mostly rocks on section A; asphalt on Berma Road

HIKING TIME 4–4.5 hours

DRIVING DISTANCE 20 miles

SEASON Year-round

ACCESS Open daily, sunrise–sunset

WHEELCHAIR TRAVERSABLE No

MAPS National Park Service, tinyurl.com /candomap

FACILITIES Restrooms, water, and phone at trailhead and off-trail at Great Falls (plus warm-season snack bar at Great Falls); restrooms near start of Berma Road and Old Angler's Inn

CONTACT Great Falls Tavern Visitor Center, 301-299-3613, nps.gov/choh; park headquarters in Sharpsburg, 301-739-4200

LOCATION Potomac, Maryland

COMMENTS There is a $10 fee to enter the park. Billy Goat Trail section A is strenuous and involves a lot of rock scrambling and good balance. Be sure to wear appropriate footwear. The hike is not recommended for small children and those with chronic medical conditions. The trail can be dangerous when wet or icy.

the falls. Before the covered stop gate, turn right at a sign for the blue-blazed Billy Goat Trail section A.

For most of its roughly 2 miles, section A follows the perimeter of Bear Island. It includes a rocky clifftop route along the Potomac's narrow, mile-long Mather Gorge. The blue blazes lead through a wild and beautiful landscape dominated by steep rocks and scraggy vegetation. Wend your way around huge boulders, over smaller ones, and past huge potholes and rockbound ponds, some with water lilies.

Between trail markers 1 and 2, you will climb a steep traverse, the most difficult part of the hike. Just after marker 2, the trail descends to a nice beach area. Continue past two small ponds as you reach marker 3. There is one more panoramic view of the river before the trail passes Sherwin Island. Eventually, after the trail curves left again, you'll reach the towpath, near the southern end of Widewater. Turn right and walk along the towpath 0.6 mile to the entrance of Billy Goat Trail section B.

This part of the hike is much easier, with only a small section of rock-hopping near Hermit Island. The 1.4-mile trail passes through a floodplain forest and along the river. Section B is the best of the three for birding, especially in the spring. Continue past the entrance to Marsden Tract Campground. When you arrive back on the towpath, turn left, heading back toward Great Falls Tavern.

A half mile up-canal (thick woods hide the Potomac here), you'll pass milepost 12 (the towpath is studded with mileposts, starting in Washington). Then, about

Billy Goat Trail: Sections A and B

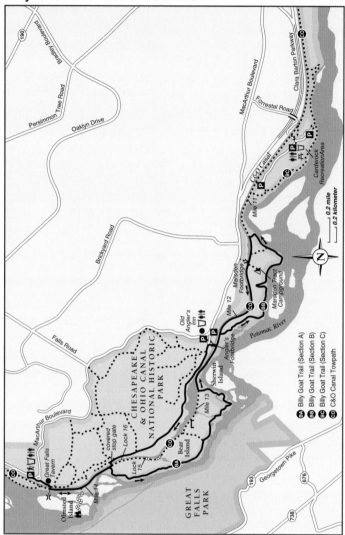

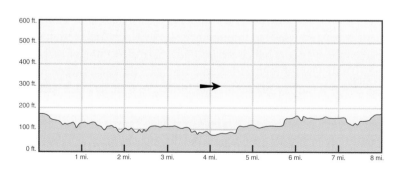

0.3 mile past milepost 12, turn right to cross the canal by footbridge and ascend some steps (off to the right is historic Old Angler's Inn); then turn left and proceed along the tree-shrouded, old, paved Berma Road. The road parallels the canal and provides great views from above in fall and winter when the trees are bare. It also connects to the Gold Mine Loop, a 1.6-mile trail around the historic Maryland Mine that dates to 1867.

Eventually, turn left and descend some steps to recross the canal on a wooden walkway. That's the upper part of a reconstructed stop gate, which was designed to divert floodwater out of the canal and into the river and is still used during floods. Descend from the walkway to rejoin the towpath (about 0.75 mile past milepost 13), and proceed up-canal. For the next half mile, look to your left for dramatic views of the river's rapids-filled side channels. Arriving at lock 20, step across a short wooden bridge spanning the canal to return to Great Falls Tavern. Connecting back to the towpath for this last section of the hike provides the most scenic views. Alternately, you can stay on the Gold Mine Loop until it ends and leads back to the visitor center.

NEARBY/RELATED ACTIVITIES

Check out the exhibits at Great Falls Tavern, and learn about the history, geology, recreation, flora, and fauna of the C&O Canal and Great Falls Park. From early April through the end of October, take a mule-drawn boat ride on the *Charles F. Mercer*. Tours given by park rangers dressed in historical clothing transport passengers back in time to the 1870s. For lunch, enjoy American cuisine (and alfresco dining in warmer weather) in a beautiful setting at Old Angler's Inn.

• •

GPS TRAILHEAD COORDINATES N39° 0.122' W77° 14.829'

> **DIRECTIONS** From the Capital Beltway (I-495), take Exit 41 toward Carderock/Great Falls 0.3 mile. Merge onto Clara Barton Parkway. Go 1.5 miles and then make a slight left onto MacArthur Boulevard. Go 3.4 miles to the entrance of the Chesapeake & Ohio Canal National Historical Park, 11710 MacArthur Blvd. NW, Potomac, Maryland.

The hike along Little Seneca Lake offers many scenic vistas.

SITUATED IN NORTHERN MONTGOMERY COUNTY, this park is an attractive locale where hikers can vigorously roam suburban parkland. It features a large lake, rolling woodlands, meadows, and a seasonal variety of views.

DESCRIPTION

Located about 21 miles northwest of Washington, Black Hill Regional Park covers 1,854 acres of rolling woodlands, meadows, and water. In fact, water is the park's dominant physical feature, with Little Seneca Lake accounting for almost a third of the acreage. The lake, the metro area's largest, clearly ranks as the multiuse park's chief attraction.

The 505-acre lake's presence makes the park doubly attractive for hikers. The irregularly shaped body of water (it resembles the head of a trident) provides one part of a fine hiking venue. The other part consists of hilly woodlands and meadows away from the lake. And the popularity of the lake and nearby recreational facilities tends to minimize traffic on the trails. For hikers, the park usually seems especially uncrowded, as most of the few other trail users are on bikes or horses.

Four decades ago, the area consisted of privately owned fields, woods, and streams. Then the metro area's water authority and Montgomery County agreed to

LENGTH 8.1 miles (with shorter options)

CONFIGURATION Out-and-back

DIFFICULTY Easy

SCENERY Woodlands, meadows, stream valleys, lake views

EXPOSURE Mostly shady; less so in winter

TRAFFIC Usually light; heavier on warm-weather weekends and holidays, especially on hiker/biker trail and near visitor center

TRAIL SURFACE Mostly pavement; some dirt and grass

HIKING TIME 2.5–3 hours

DRIVING DISTANCE 37 miles

SEASON Year-round

ACCESS Open daily, 6 a.m.–sunset, March–October (7 a.m.–sunset in other months)

WHEELCHAIR TRAVERSABLE No

MAPS Montgomery Parks, montgomery parks.org

CONTACT Black Hill Visitor Center (open Wednesday–Friday, 11 a.m.–5 p.m., and Saturday–Sunday, 11 a.m.–6 p.m.), 301-972-3476

FACILITIES Restrooms and water at visitor center, boat dock, parking lot 5, and picnic shelters (warm season); phones at entrance kiosk and visitor center

LOCATION Boyds, Maryland

COMMENTS The park has a great visitor center with exhibits and friendly staff. Montgomery County runs regularly scheduled naturalist-guided programs for kids and adults.

create a dual-use emergency water-supply reservoir and park. Little Seneca Creek was dammed, stream valleys filled up, and farmers left. When it opened in 1987, the park was still enveloped in farmland. But since then, residential development spreading west from Germantown has reached the park boundary.

However, some two decades of protective park status have helped Black Hill nurture a rich population of plants and animals. Woodlands dominate, with oaks, hickories, beeches, maples, tulip trees, and conifers being seasonally complemented by bloom-laden bushes and wildflowers. Deer are plentiful, as are smaller animals. Seasonally, myriad birds contribute color, song, insect control, and seed dispersal. In winter, fish-hungry bald eagles and ospreys enhance the lake view.

The 8.1-mile hike route uses the park's main trail network, following the paved Black Hill Trail from the visitor center to the southern end of Little Seneca Lake. The trails are not blazed but are generally well signposted (except at the hike's start). Navigating them is pretty easy; anytime you reach an intersection, just turn right.

To get started, face the visitor center, and take the paved trail on the left. You will see three paths, which may seem confusing. One leads to the lake and boat rentals, another leads to a picnic area, and the third one heads uphill away from the lake. Take the trail that is farthest to the left and heads toward the street. As you begin the trail, you'll pass restrooms on the right, and then head down the hill, where you will pass a sign for the Black Hill Trail. The trail begins along Lake Ridge Drive, follows the creek, and then hugs the shore of the lake for a little more than 2 miles.

Black Hill Regional Park

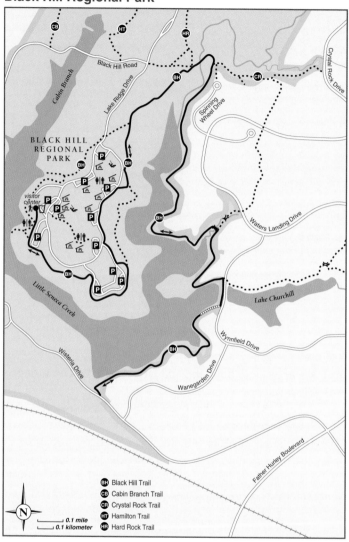

BLACK HILL
REGIONAL
PARK

*visitor
center*

Black Hill Road

Cabin Branch

Lake Ridge Drive

Spinning
Wheel Drive

Crystal Rock Drive

Waters Landing Drive

Little Seneca Creek

Lake Churchill

Wynnfield Drive

Wisteria Drive

Wanegarden Drive

Father Hurley Boulevard

N

0.1 mile
0.1 kilometer

BH Black Hill Trail
CB Cabin Branch Trail
CP Crystal Rock Trail
HT Hamilton Trail
HR Hard Rock Trail

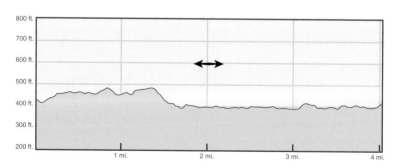

When you come to an intersection with the natural-surface trail, make a right to stay on the paved Black Hill Trail. You will pass by the Parcourse Fitness Circuit, a series of fitness stations that you can use to improve your cardiovascular strength and conditioning if you have some extra energy.

The path is a hiker/biker trail that's wide enough for two people to easily walk side by side; hikers should stay alert for bikers and move over to let them pass. When the trail intersects with Crystal Rock Trail, turn right to stay on Black Hill Trail. You will come to a long stretch of chain-link fence that runs along the trail next to the woods. Follow the bridge across the stream on the boardwalk. The trail goes up a hill, and you'll pass a sign for Waters' Mill. In the 1780s, the Waters family owned acreage here known as the William and Mary Tract. Around 1810, Zachariah Waters built a gristmill on a portion of the tract to process grain, lumber, and flax seed. The mill ceased operation around 1895. Remains of the property are located along Little Seneca Creek.

At the next intersection, make a right to stay on the trail. When you come to a bench and a bridge, turn right to go over the bridge, turn right again, and proceed on the trail toward the lake. As you reach Wynnfield Drive, cross the street carefully and stay on the trail following the edge of the lake. The trail continues a short way, ending at Wisteria Drive. Turn around and hike back the way you came.

To shorten this hike and maximize the views, park and begin your hike near shelter J, parking lot 9 (past the visitor center) along Lake Ridge Drive.

NEARBY/RELATED ACTIVITIES

At any time of year, explore the visitor center and linger with binoculars on the center's always-open observation deck for panoramic views of the lake. In winter, watch for bald eagles and ospreys. In warm weather, explore the lake by rental boat (available Wednesday–Sunday); call 301-972-6157. Follow the Black Hill Water Trail and take a tour of Little Seneca Lake in a canoe or kayak, and learn more about the ecology, plants, and wildlife around the lake. Following the water trail markers takes 3–5 hours.

• •

GPS TRAILHEAD COORDINATES N39° 11.543' W77° 17.749'

> **DIRECTIONS** From the junction of the Capital Beltway (I-495) and I-270 Spur in Maryland, head northwest on I-270 (toward Frederick) about 18.5 miles. Get off at Exit 18 and turn left onto Clarksburg Road (MD 121). Proceed generally south about 1.6 miles. Then turn left onto West Old Baltimore Road. Go east 1 mile, and turn right into the park. Take Lake Ridge Drive 2 miles to the visitor center parking lot. Arrive early to beat the crowds during warm months.

14 BROOKSIDE GARDENS AND WHEATON REGIONAL PARK

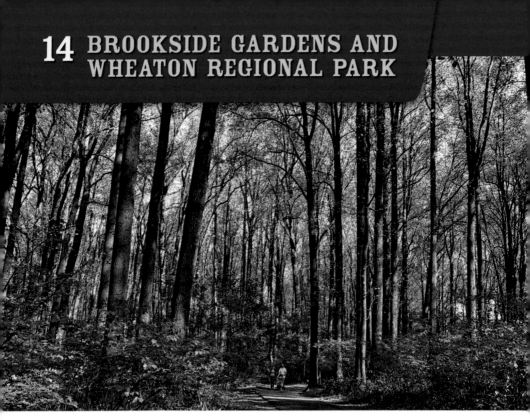

Wheaton Regional Park has a tall canopy forest perfect for shady walks on stroller-friendly paved paths.

BROOKSIDE GARDENS and Wheaton Regional Park are two of Montgomery County's most popular parks, giving hikers opportunities to see a variety of attractions while enjoying the natural environment. Montgomery Parks continues to expand and improve the facilities and gardens, and it seems like there's always something new to see.

DESCRIPTION

Brookside Gardens is truly a treasure. Founded by the Maryland National Capital Park and Planning Commission in 1965, the property encompasses 54 acres, with 32 acres of cultivated gardens, and has more than 400,000 visitors each year. The European landscape architect was inspired by garden styles found in Germany and Switzerland. The gardens are like separate rooms with different themes, including a wedding gazebo, an azalea walk, an aquatic garden, a Japanese teahouse, a rose garden, and a winter garden. The conservatory complex was installed in 1969–1971 with tropical plants and today houses the annual Wings of Fancy Live Butterfly Exhibit during the summer and the Garden of Lights during the winter holidays. In 2004 a reflection terrace was dedicated to the victims of the 2002 sniper shootings in Montgomery County.

Begin your hike by parking at the Brookside Gardens Visitor Center, and ask for a trail map at the information desk. Walk outside the visitor center door, past the

LENGTH 4.4 miles (with shorter options)

CONFIGURATION Loop

DIFFICULTY Easy–moderate

SCENERY Forested hills and valleys, gardens, playground, miniature train, fountains, carousel

EXPOSURE Partially shady; much less so in winter

TRAFFIC Medium–heavy on weekends and holidays

TRAIL SURFACE Gravel, paved, dirt

HIKING TIME 3 hours (with time to check out the conservatory complex, gardens, playground, and historic sites)

DRIVING DISTANCE 26 miles

SEASON Year-round, but best in summer, spring, and fall

ACCESS Grounds are open sunrise–sunset; gardens are open 9 a.m.–5 p.m.; conservatory complex is open 10 a.m.–5 p.m.

WHEELCHAIR TRAVERSABLE Partially

MAPS Montgomery Parks, montgomeryparks .org, tinyurl.com/wheatonparkmap

FACILITIES Visitor center at Brookside Gardens; water fountains and restrooms at Wheaton Regional Park

CONTACT 301-962-1400, tinyurl.com /brooksidegardens

LOCATION Wheaton, Maryland

COMMENTS These parks provide all-day entertainment, so expect to spend lots of time. During the holidays, Brookside Gardens has an elaborate ornamental light display.

children's garden, and take a right on the asphalt path that traverses a meadow. The Japanese gardens are to your left, and you'll see a pagoda and picturesque Pine Lake. Continue down the asphalt trail until you see a metal fence that opens into Wheaton Regional Park. Walk through the gate, following the trail into the forest.

At the first intersection, take a right and begin the loop. You'll pass the Sligo Creek Park playground and picnic areas of Wheaton Regional Park. This section of the trail can accommodate a stroller, wheelchair, or skateboard. When you come to a fork in the road, you'll be in the playground. Check out the many accessible playground activities, including a man-made Blue Hill, swings and slides, picnic areas, and Wheaton Regional Nature Center. Walk behind the carousel and train station toward the parking lot. The trailhead is on the other end of this asphalt parking lot.

Continue on the Wheaton Regional Trail, following the white blazes. Next, you'll cross Henderson Avenue, a service road leading to a neighborhood. Stay on the asphalt trail, bypassing the sign for the Sligo Creek trailhead. Cross a small creek, and then make a left on the trail. At the guardrail make a left, continuing into the woods. The trees here consist of mostly beech, oak, tulip poplar, cherry, and sycamore. Listen closely, and you may hear a woodpecker at work.

When the trail jogs left, you'll see athletic fields and tennis courts. To your left, in the distance, you'll see the Wheaton Sports Pavilion. Cross this road, and at the next intersection, follow the Arcola Trail and signs pointing toward the nature center. At the next intersection, you'll see a wooded connector trail (this is the end of the paved trail). If you want to shorten the hike, this is a good time to walk 0.5 mile

Brookside Gardens and Wheaton Regional Park

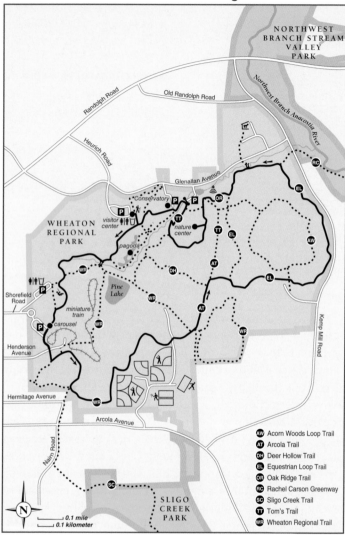

NORTHWEST BRANCH STREAM VALLEY PARK

Randolph Road
Old Randolph Road
Northwest Branch Anacostia River

Heurich Road

Glenallan Avenue

Conservatory

WHEATON REGIONAL PARK

visitor center

nature center

pagoda

Pine Lake

miniature train

Shorefield Road

carousel

Henderson Avenue

Hermitage Avenue

Arcola Avenue

Nairn Road

Kemp Mill Road

SLIGO CREEK PARK

N

0.1 mile
0.1 kilometer

- **AW** Acorn Woods Loop Trail
- **AT** Arcola Trail
- **DH** Deer Hollow Trail
- **EL** Equestrian Loop Trail
- **OR** Oak Ridge Trail
- **RC** Rachel Carson Greenway
- **SC** Sligo Creek Trail
- **TT** Tom's Trail
- **WR** Wheaton Regional Trail

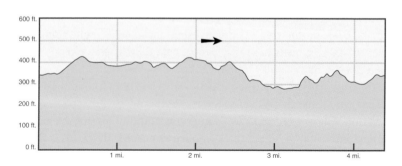

600 ft.
500 ft.
400 ft.
300 ft.
200 ft.
100 ft.
0 ft.

1 mi.   2 mi.   3 mi.   4 mi.

on the Arcola Trail to the Brookside Gardens Visitor Center. If you wish to continue, follow the blue blazes on the dirt trail.

Pass an intersection for Deer Hollow Trail, and at the dead end, turn right and begin following the Equestrian Trail Loop at least 1 mile. This dirt trail skirts the perimeter of Wheaton Regional, so you often come close to Kemp Mill Road and then Glenallan Avenue. Follow the blue blazes as the trail undulates through thick, pristine woodland.

After you've made your way around the loop, you'll come to some stairs and the beginning of the Oak Ridge Trail that loops around the nature center. Pass an amphitheater and a sign designating the Underground Railroad. You'll see Brookside Gardens Nature Center to your right and a clearing with a log cabin and outdoor smokehouse up the hill on the left. This is the homestead of the Harper family, built in 1870. The family was part of a freed-slave community called Jonesville, just north of Poolesville in Montgomery County. The heirs of the second owner, Henry Willard, donated it to the Montgomery Parks Department. The cabin was dismantled, moved, and reassembled here. Examine the Harper homestead, and walk through the grounds of the nature center on the self-guided Nature Trail loop. Look for the signs pointing toward the Brookside Gardens conservatory and visitor center.

Finding your way back to the visitor center is a bit confusing. Take Tom's Trail loop, passing the aquatic gardens and fountain. You'll see signs for a lizard sanctuary and information about various native plants, such as the spicebush and gum tree. After following the self-guided loop, turn right and follow signs to the conservatory and visitor center. Cross the bridge and walk through the gate. Walk across a boardwalk, pass the conservatory, and head into the stone gardens. Walk up the stone steps toward the pavilion and back to the visitor center.

NEARBY/RELATED ACTIVITIES

For kids, the park has an extensive playground, a miniature train, and a 1915 carousel (the train and carousel operate on weekends only in April and September and daily May–August). There's also a dog park for your furry friends. The Wheaton Riding Stables are just across Glenallan Avenue. The athletic complex is a fun place to play tennis, in-line skate, or ice-skate. Downtown Wheaton has a cornucopia of fabulous ethnic restaurants, especially Asian and Peruvian. Westfield Wheaton Mall has a movie theater, restaurants, and lots of shopping.

• •

GPS TRAILHEAD COORDINATES N39° 03.492' W77° 02.229'

DIRECTIONS From the Capital Beltway (I-495), take Exit 31A to go north on Georgia Avenue/MD 97 toward Wheaton. Drive 3 miles to Randolph Road; turn right. At the second traffic light, turn right onto Glenallan Avenue.

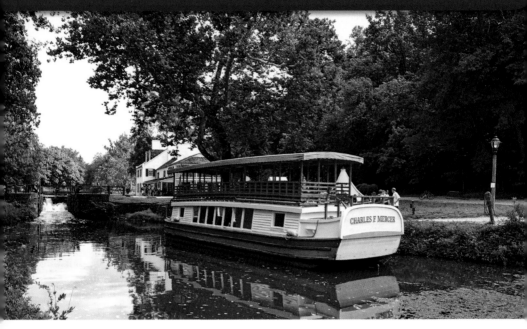

After visiting the Great Falls Tavern Visitor Center, take a ride on a boat down the C&O Canal.

SCENERY, EXERCISE, AND GLIMPSES OF HISTORY—the C&O Canal Towpath has it all, and it is almost completely level. This close-in segment in Montgomery County features a waterfall, a visitor center, and a towpath used by mules to pull barges in the 1700s.

DESCRIPTION

The Chesapeake & Ohio Canal National Historical Park ranks as one of the area's prime recreational resources, although its storied history includes nearly being paved over to develop a highway to downtown Washington, D.C. Today, the National Park Service oversees this scenic stretch of land and has been successful in preserving the land, flora, fauna, and many historic sites along 185 miles of the Potomac River's left bank. The restored canal towpath is now a popular multiuse trail, with detours where hikers can savor nature and even find solitude. The landscape you see today has been shaped by both natural and man-made forces.

The C&O Canal had its origins in a grand ambition voiced by Thomas Jefferson, George Washington, and other early American leaders. Their goal was to make the Potomac River navigable and link it to the Ohio River valley. The Patowmack Company, chartered in 1785 with George Washington as its first president, announced it

LENGTH 5.4 miles (with shorter and longer options)

CONFIGURATION Modified out-and-back with detour

DIFFICULTY Easy

SCENERY Water, woodlands, thundering waterfalls

EXPOSURE Mostly open

TRAFFIC Steady stream of visitors; heaviest on warm-weather weekends and holidays

TRAIL SURFACE Hard-packed dirt on towpath; dirt, rocks, and roots on side trails

HIKING TIME 3 hours

DRIVING DISTANCE 20 miles

SEASON Year-round

ACCESS Visitor center is open daily, 10 a.m.–4 p.m. Trail is open sunrise–sunset.

WHEELCHAIR TRAVERSABLE Yes, on towpath

MAPS National Park Service, tinyurl.com /candomap

FACILITIES Restrooms and water at Great Falls Tavern Visitor Center and at Old Angler's Inn; restrooms and changing room near start of Berma Road and Old Angler's Inn

CONTACT Great Falls Tavern Visitor Center, open 9 a.m.–4:30 p.m.; 301-767-3714; nps.gov /grfa. Old Angler's Inn, open 11:30 a.m.–2:30 p.m. and 5:30–9:30 p.m.; 301-365-2425; oldanglersinn.com

LOCATION Potomac, Maryland

COMMENTS There is a $10 fee to enter the park. Trail can be slippery when wet or icy.

would clear a channel and build skirting canals around the rapids. Immigrants were welcomed to do the heavy lifting of many physical obstacles that hampered progress. It took nearly 20 years just to complete the canals. The channel was never cleared completely, and boat travel was severely limited by fluctuating water levels. The Patowmack Company eventually collapsed.

The Chesapeake & Ohio Canal Company, launched in 1828, inherited its predecessor's charter and property. Its plan was to stay out of the river and build an on-land canal dotted with locks and paralleled by a towpath for the mules and horses that would provide the motive power for the boats. The canal was not finished until 1850—eight years after the Baltimore & Ohio Railroad had reached Cumberland—so the canal was already largely obsolete commercially. The Civil War and recurrent floods further damaged the canal and its toll-based business. After a devastating 1889 flood, the waterway was bought by the B&O. The C&O Canal remained in sporadic and local use until 1924, when another flood led the B&O to abandon it. In 1938 the railroad gave it to the federal government to settle a $2 million debt.

The National Park Service managed to restore the canal's lower 22 miles before World War II intervened but did little else for a long time thereafter. In 1954 a public campaign launched by Supreme Court justice and outdoorsman William O. Douglas saved the canal route from being paved over as a parkway. In solidarity, US Attorney General Robert Kennedy invited his press corps to accompany him on a 50-mile hike from Great Falls, Maryland, to Harpers Ferry, West Virginia. Both of these influential

C&O Canal Towpath: Great Falls to Old Angler's Inn with Olmsted Island

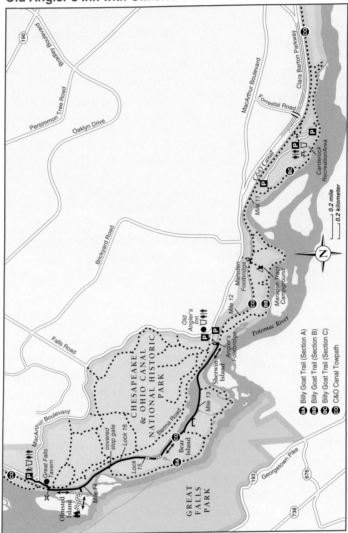

leaders brought attention to the canal's natural beauty. Congress made the property a national monument in 1961 and a national historical park in 1971.

Located just outside the beltway, on MacArthur Boulevard, you'll find ample parking, but prepare to pay an entrance fee of $10 per vehicle. Of all the hikes on the C&O Canal, this section is probably the most popular because of its access to the thundering cascade of whitewater called Great Falls. To view Great Falls Overlook from the Maryland side, you will walk along man-made boardwalks and concrete bridges through the wetlands to Olmsted Island. Some crossing points may be a bit scary, but the effort is worth it for this panoramic view of the Potomac's mightiest waterfall.

After parking, find your way to the Great Falls Tavern Visitor Center to check out the museum and get a map. Rangers are usually available to answer questions about the hiking trails. Originally, in the 1820s, the building was a lockhouse where canal operators lowered and raised the locks for canal boats carrying coal upstream from Maryland's western counties south to Georgetown. The visitor center has restrooms and weekend bike rentals and is where visitors may pay a $5–$8 fee for a mule-drawn boat ride on the canal. The *Charles F. Mercer* canal boat operates on weekends from the end of March until October 30 at 11:30 a.m., 1:30 p.m., and 3 p.m. (but it's worth checking before you go). On some weekends you might see living history encampments with reenactors dressed in Civil War uniforms.

The trailhead crosses over a bridge just past the visitor center and proceeds south on the towpath. After lock 18, you will see the entrance to Olmsted Island. Follow this path into the fairylike woods, where boulders are covered with lichens, hardwood trees are decorated with moss, and lush grasses and thistles grow. As you continue to pass over the protected wetlands on the boardwalk, you'll come to two precarious concrete bridges where you'll cross over chutes of swiftly moving currents of water tumbling over steep rocks. After that excitement, prepare to walk single file down narrow passages until you reach the Great Falls Overlook. Across the Potomac River, you may see your fellow hikers on the Virginia side. In good weather, kayakers enjoy playing around at the base of Great Falls. To return to the trail, retrace your steps.

After you return to the towpath, turn right. Just after lock 17, you will pass the entrance to Billy Goat Trail section A (Hike 12, page 68). The arduous and very popular trail requires scrambling over angled rocks and boulders for 1.7 miles. It's quite challenging, especially when there are lots of people, but it offers breathtaking views and a great workout.

For this towpath hike, you will continue walking on the dirt towpath, all the while making way for bikes by staying to the right. The towpath is a favorite for parents taking the kids for a stroll and dog owners giving their dogs a nice stretch. If you come here on weekday mornings, you might find groups of high-school kids collecting water samples for their biology class.

At lock 15, the trail becomes a boardwalk. Around this point, the canal opens up and widens to an expansive view. This section is called Widewater, and there are two shady benches if you want to rest for a minute and enjoy the view. Look to the right, on the Potomac River side, for ponds where turtles sun themselves on fallen tree trunks. A little farther down from mile marker 13, you'll see another entrance to the Billy Goat Trail section A.

It's time to turn around when you get to a wooden bridge, which leads to the rustic Old Angler's Inn restaurant, parking lot, and bathrooms. This is where most of the kayakers come to put in. You can either turn around and retrace your steps, or in fine weather you can go up and have a snack or meal at the restaurant's outdoor patio. If you prefer not to retrace your steps, take the Berma Road Trail on the eastern side of the C&O Canal. Berma Road is a 1.5-mile return trip to Great Falls Tavern Visitor Center.

NEARBY/RELATED ACTIVITIES

Check out the museum inside the Great Falls Tavern Visitor Center. Take a canal boat ride (when in season). Extend your hike to watch the rock climbers in Carderock's Mather Gorge (Hike 16, page 85). Hike one of the challenging Billy Goat Trails (Hike 12, page 68), on which you'll scramble over rocks and find breathtaking views of the wild Potomac River. Head to Potomac Village to grab a bite at one of its many restaurants and coffee shops.

• •

GPS TRAILHEAD COORDINATES N39° 0.122' W77° 14.829'

> **DIRECTIONS** From the Capital Beltway (I-495), take Exit 41 west toward Carderock/Great Falls 0.3 mile. Merge onto Clara Barton Parkway. Go 1.5 miles and then make a slight left onto MacArthur Boulevard. Go 3.4 miles to the entrance of the Chesapeake & Ohio Canal National Historical Park, 11710 MacArthur Blvd. NW, Potomac, Maryland.

The historic canal used a system of locks to change the water levels and move boats along the Potomac.

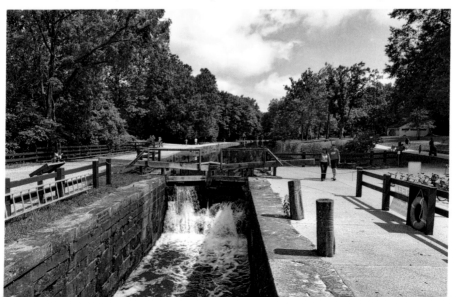

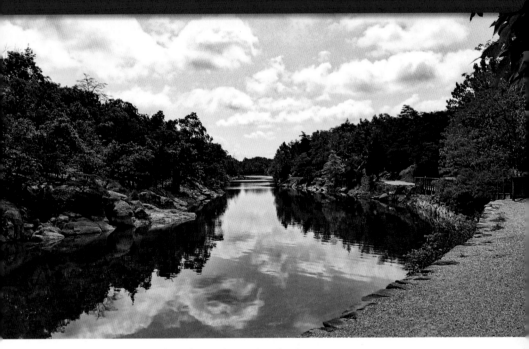

Widewater is a scenic spot where the canal expands and makes a turn.

THE C&O CANAL TOWPATH offers multiple sections of trails, each with its own unique features. Here, the dynamic rock faces at Carderock are a favorite place for local climbers, and this section is one of the best urban cliff areas in the eastern United States. Old Angler's Inn is a historic restaurant and is a popular meeting place for kayakers who launch here.

DESCRIPTION

The hike begins across the canal from Old Angler's Inn, a restaurant with a storied history. This site was a common meeting place for American Indians of the Algonquin Nation. During the 1700s, European settlers maintained a post for traveling traders where Old Angler's Inn now stands. Just a few miles from here, Captain John Smith made camp on his canoe trip up the Potomac River, referred to as the Patawomeck River back in 1608. George Washington crossed the river near this landmark during the French and Indian Wars on his way to fight the French at Fort Duquesne. President John Quincy Adams marked the same site when he shoveled dirt at the groundbreaking for the Chesapeake & Ohio Canal. In 1860, the inn opened, offering respite for people traveling from the capital to rural Maryland.

LENGTH 4.7 miles (with shorter and longer options)

CONFIGURATION Out-and-back

DIFFICULTY Easy

SCENERY Water, woodlands

EXPOSURE Mostly open

TRAFFIC Light on weekdays and in the winter; heavier on warm-weather evenings, weekends, and holidays

TRAIL SURFACE Hard-packed dirt on towpath; asphalt on Clara Barton Parkway; dirt, rocks, and roots on side trails

HIKING TIME 2 hours (with a stop to watch the climbers)

DRIVING DISTANCE 18 miles

SEASON Year-round

ACCESS Open daily, sunrise–sunset

WHEELCHAIR TRAVERSABLE Yes, on the towpath

MAPS National Park Service, tinyurl.com/candomap

FACILITIES Restrooms and water at Old Angler's Inn and Carderock Recreation Area

CONTACT Old Angler's Inn, open 11:30 a.m.–2:30 p.m. and 5:30–9:30 p.m.; 301-365-2425; oldanglersinn.com. Carderock Recreation Area, 301-767-3703, nps.gov/choh

LOCATION Potomac, Maryland

COMMENTS Trail can be slippery when wet or icy.

During the Civil War, couriers exchanging messages between both the Union and Confederate Armies would often stop at Old Angler's Inn for a meal or to rest. President Theodore Roosevelt enjoyed fishing around Widewater, a naturally formed link of the canal that is just steps from the inn. In 1957, John Reges bought the inn for his wife, Olympia, who restored its historic charm and eventually opened the popular restaurant. Old Angler's Inn became a favorite dining spot for Washingtonians, and today the Reges family continues to operate the restaurant, with its rustic outdoor patio.

Park on MacArthur Boulevard or in the gravel parking lot across the street from Old Angler's Inn. Walk down through the trees to a bridge that crosses the C&O Canal to the towpath. Turn left and head south on the towpath (toward Washington, D.C.). If you turn right, you're headed toward Great Falls Tavern Visitor Center (see page 80).

The hike begins in a swampy part of the canal that is also thick with brush. Just a few steps into the hike, you'll see an entrance to Billy Goat Trail section B. This is typically the end of this 1.4-mile trail that follows the contours of the Potomac River shoreline (see page 68 for trail information). Continue walking on the towpath as the canal widens. You'll see that many trees have fallen from the hillside into the water, and you can imagine how difficult it must have been to construct this canal in the late 1700s before there was heavy construction equipment to dig trenches and lift boulders.

In a little less than a mile, you'll come upon Marsden Bridge at the entrance to Marsden Tract Campground. This is a recreation area with multiple campsites used by Scout troops and local groups. After that, the thick brush opens up on the riverside, and you'll catch glimpses of the huge rock faces that attract rock-climbing

C&O Canal Towpath: Old Angler's Inn to Carderock Recreation Area

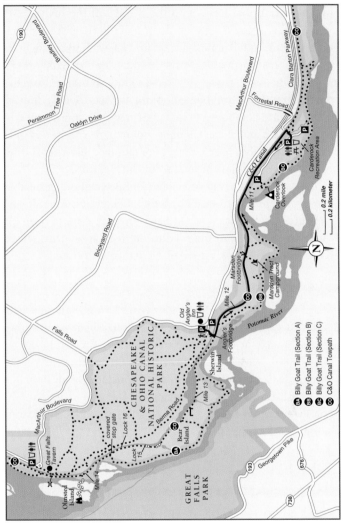

enthusiasts from all over. You'll also see Vaso Island and, if it's winter, maybe out to Turkey Island where the Potomac River pushes into the land.

Just after mile marker 11, you'll pass the entrance to Billy Goat Trail section C. The trail eerily disappears down the hill and into the woods. For a more challenging hike than the towpath, you can follow this 1.6-mile section to the west of the towpath, a scenic woodland trek along the edge of a side channel and then a main channel. It has its ups and downs, but it's a lot easier than sections A and B. It is also harder to follow, so keep an eye out for the blue blazes.

Back on the towpath, you'll come to the entrance of the Potomac Gorge with its parking lot and a trail that heads into the woods off the towpath. Follow that trail toward the river, and you'll arrive at the top of the steep faces of volcanic rock that make up Carderock. You'll almost always find a few climbers there, belaying up these steep boulders. It's worthwhile to spend some time watching them in action. The 25- to 60-foot-high, west-facing cliffs have routes that range from easy to moderate. The quartz knobs and nubbins allow for novice-friendly moves and solid handholds. The cliffs are composed of metamorphic rock transformed by heat and pressure from mudstone and shale. Climbers come here year-round, and although there are restrooms here, they aren't always operational. Just a short distance north is the Carderock Pavilion, with picnic and restroom facilities.

Return to the towpath the way you came, and you can either head back to Old Angler's trailhead or continue toward Carderock Recreation Area. If you continue, you'll pass the water treatment plant until the towpath crosses over Clara Barton Parkway. If you wish, walk down the road to the recreation area, where there are picnic tables, barbecue grills, and a good place to throw a Frisbee.

NEARBY/RELATED ACTIVITIES

Bring a picnic and enjoy Carderock Recreation Area. Extend your hike to begin at the C&O Canal Visitor Center, where you can take a canal boat ride (in the summer), see an original lockhouse, or walk to the overlook on Olmsted Island to see Great Falls (Hike 15, page 80). Just a few miles away, pick up healthy treats at the Bethesda Co-op. Take the kids to play at nearby Cabin John Park, with its miniature train rides, climbing installations, and ice-skating rink. Drive to Scott's Run Nature Preserve in nearby Virginia to see the C&O Canal and Carderock Cliffs from the other side of the Potomac River (Hike 38, page 178).

• •

GPS TRAILHEAD COORDINATES N38° 58.894' W77° 13.686'

> **DIRECTIONS** Take I-495 to Exit 41 west toward Carderock/Great Falls. At the T intersection, turn left on MacArthur Boulevard. Go about 1 mile until you come to Old Angler's Inn at 10801 MacArthur Blvd. Use street parking or the lot across from Old Angler's.

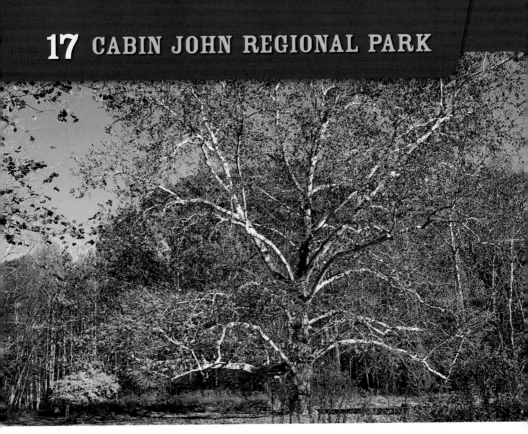

Under the shade of this ancient sycamore tree, you'll find benches for picnics and gatherings.

A FAVORITE DESTINATION FOR KIDS AND DOG WALKERS, Cabin John Regional Park encompasses the Locust Grove Nature Center, a miniature train, Bethesda Big Train 1A Pro Baseball Stadium, a huge playground, an ice rink, and other recreational facilities. This trail originates at Tuckerman Lane and ends on Democracy Boulevard.

DESCRIPTION

Cabin John Regional Park is part of the Cabin John Stream Valley Trail. The park was designed to provide recreation and protect this tributary of the Potomac River. The entire length of the Cabin John Stream Valley Trail stretches 8.8 miles from Tuckerman Lane to the C&O Canal Towpath. The trails cross multiple high-traffic roads, so we limited our hike to the northern section with no major road crossings.

When European settlers first arrived in the lowlands of what is now Cabin John, they found the Susquehanna tribe. Other American Indians who lived in the area were the Piscataway and the Seneca. Lord Baltimore was the proprietor of Maryland in the middle of the 17th century, making land grants to settlers who wanted to farm tobacco. During the building of the C&O Canal in the 1820s, more Europeans

LENGTH 3 miles (with longer and shorter options)

CONFIGURATION Modified loop

DIFFICULTY Easy

SCENERY Stream views, forest, nature center

EXPOSURE Mostly shady; less so in winter

TRAFFIC Usually light

TRAIL SURFACE Hard-packed dirt, rocky and rooty

HIKING TIME 1 hour

DRIVING DISTANCE 28 miles

SEASON Year-round

ACCESS Open daily, sunrise–sunset; road within park opens 8 a.m., closes 1 hour before sunset

WHEELCHAIR TRAVERSABLE No

MAPS Montgomery Parks, montgomery parks.org

FACILITIES Water, phone at nature center

CONTACT 301-765-8650 or montgomery parks.org

LOCATION Bethesda, Maryland

COMMENTS No fees to park or hike; some bicycles use these paths but not often.

moved here seeking work on the canal and later on the Washington Aqueduct in the 1850s and 1860s.

Although there are many versions of this story, and nothing is fully documented, the name Cabin John may come from a hermit named John who had a cabin at the Union Arch Bridge. The Cabin John Citizens Association historians say the name may be derived from Captain John Smith, founder of Jamestown and the first to map the Potomac River near Cabin John. Around 1912, the American Land Company bought a large tract of land in Cabin John and divided it into residential lots. In the 1940s the federal government built 20 houses for black workers, and many of these families remain in the community as important voices of leadership.

The trail contains diverse flora—a thick forest of oak, beech, tulip trees, and one of the area's largest sycamores. Despite heavy year-round use, the land remains wild and natural, even a bit hilly. To begin your hike, park on the west side of the parking lot in front of the Cabin John Indoor Tennis Center. Look for the Pine Ridge trail-head at the edge of the parking lot, and enter the forest. The natural-surface trail is at times uneven with roots; it's marked with white blazes. At the end of Pine Ridge, turn right to follow the Cabin John Trail.

Cabin John Creek parallels the path on the left. The white blazes are prominent and easy to observe. You'll pass the tennis court structures up the hill on the right side. At the intersection, turn left at the wooden signpost to remain on the Cabin John Trail. Here you'll come to a clearing in the forest with a few benches and campfire around a 200-year-old sycamore tree. The trunk is approximately 144 inches wide and 85 feet tall. The lateral branches extend majestically over the field.

Right after the sycamore tree, you'll come to a sandy beach where you can walk down to the stream. You'll pass a signpost indicating the Tulip Tree Trail. If you want

Cabin John Regional Park

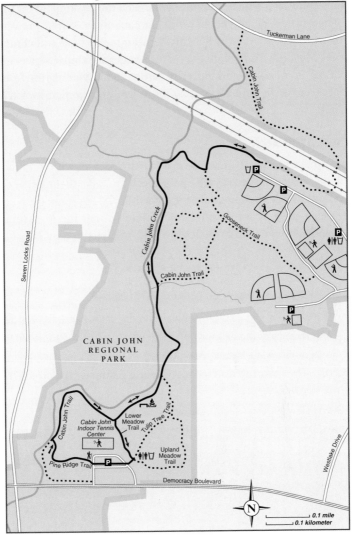

to add some distance and climb to your hike, follow the loop that meanders up the hill and meets the Upland Meadow Trail. For this hike, we stayed on the Cabin John Trail. After this intersection, you'll cross a small stream on a wooden bridge. Cross a second streambed, and then the trail splits. Turn to the left to continue to parallel the stream. At this point, the trail widens, and you get very close to the shoreline. Lots of huge fallen trees entice people to walk across, but please use extreme caution. When the power lines are visible about 100 yards away, turn right to loop back at the next fork.

Continue following blue blazes until you reach the parking lot for the baseball diamond. Then turn back and begin retracing your steps. When you see the signpost pointing to the Locust Grove Nature Center, make a left and climb the stairs on the Lower Meadow Trail. Note the mature majestic white oak trees surrounding the building, mini pond, and butterfly garden. After visiting the Locust Grove Nature Center, cross the asphalt parking lot in front of the tennis court to return to your vehicle.

NEARBY/RELATED ACTIVITIES

Spend some time exploring the Locust Grove Nature Center with its indoor oak tree exhibit and live snakes. If the kids are up for more fun, take them to the Cabin John Park playground to ride the miniature train, feed Porky Pig some trash, and try out some slides. Also close by are Westfield Montgomery Mall and the ArcLight movie theater (connected to the mall), which shows lots of first-run movies.

• •

GPS TRAILHEAD COORDINATES N39° 01.436' W77° 09.549'

DIRECTIONS From the Capital Beltway (I-495), take Exit 38 (I-270 North Spur), and then take the exit for Democracy Boulevard West toward Westfield Montgomery Mall. Pass Bells Mill Road on the left, and the parking lot for Locust Grove and Cabin John Indoor Tennis Center will be on your right.

Take a walk down to the creek, and enjoy a break from hectic urban life.

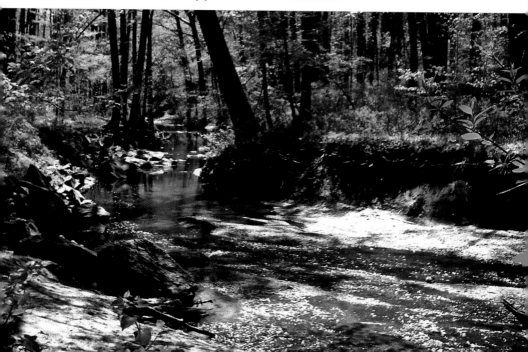

18 COSCA REGIONAL PARK

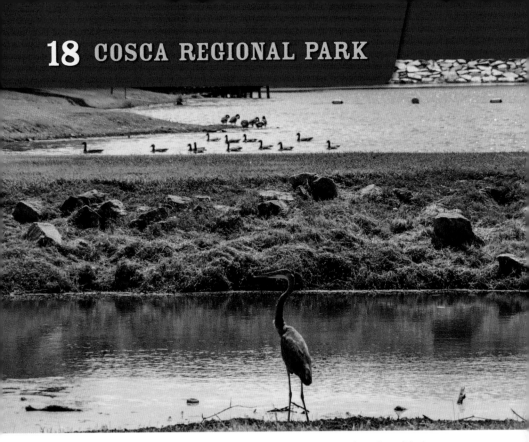

Lake Cosca attracts birds such as the great blue heron, Canada geese, and a variety of ducks.

WITH MORE THAN 690 ACRES located in southern Prince George's County, Cosca Regional Park features recreational areas and a nature center that offers a variety of interpretive programs hosted by park naturalists. Families can enjoy an easy stroll around the lake with a stop for a picnic and time to play on the playground, while more adventurous hikers may access the 3.7-mile green trail west of the lake.

DESCRIPTION

Louise F. Cosca Regional Park—one of only two hiking venues in this book named for women (see page 101 for the other)—is a small gem of a little-known nature preserve that lies near Clinton, in suburban southern Prince George's County. When opened in 1967, it was called Clinton Regional Park and was surrounded by farmlands. It was later renamed Louise F. Cosca Regional Park in memory of a member of the Maryland–National Capital Park and Planning Commission who had played a key role in its creation. Today, although some farms remain, houses abound along the park's perimeter, and the park is best known for its playing fields, man-made lake, nature center, and other amenities. Nevertheless, the park is maintained mostly

LENGTH 1.2 miles (longer options available)

CONFIGURATION Modified loop

DIFFICULTY Easy

SCENERY Rolling woodlands, lake views, stream valleys

EXPOSURE Mostly shady; less so in winter

TRAFFIC Usually light–very light; heavier close to nature center, lake, and picnic areas and on warm-weather weekends and holidays

TRAIL SURFACE Dirt and pavement, grass

HIKING TIME 1 hour

DRIVING DISTANCE 16 miles

SEASON Year-round

ACCESS Open daily, 7:30 a.m.–sunset, Clearwater Nature Center open Monday–Saturday, 8:30 a.m.–5 p.m., and Sunday, 11 a.m.–4 p.m.

WHEELCHAIR TRAVERSABLE Partially

MAPS An outdated map is available at the nature center.

FACILITIES Restrooms and water inside nature center; warm-season-only restrooms and snack bar at boathouse; warm-season-only restrooms at pavilion and off-trail at camping area; water at picnic area

CONTACT Park, 301-868-1397; nature center, 301-699-2544

LOCATION Clinton, Maryland

COMMENTS Park entrance gates close at sunset. Avoid the red trail, as it is not well maintained. Be aware that the trail map available at the nature center is outdated. The orange trail is not on the map.

as a nature preserve of woodlands where savvy hikers can enjoy nature, exercise, and solitude year-round.

This hike consists of an easy 1.2-mile loop around the lake. Beginning at the nature center parking lot, look for the trailhead with signs for the blue, green, orange, and red trails. Go down the steps, cross the entrance to the red trail, and continue straight. Turn left and follow the signs to the blue trail. When you see a view of the lake, cross the grass and stay left to follow the sand-and-dirt trail along the western edge of the man-made Lake Cosca. The woods are deciduous, with a scattering of pines and hollies. Wildflowers dapple the woods with color over three seasons. Migratory songbirds do the same in spring. Oaks, hickories, beeches, maples, tulip trees, and gums add to the park's palette in the fall. Deer and squirrels are the most frequently seen four-footed creatures, but others are also present.

If you're there on a warm-season weekend or holiday, you'll probably see boaters and other visitors, as well as mostly domesticated geese, ducks, and herons. As you reach the northern end of the lake, you may depart to the left on the green trail if you'd like to extend your excursion. The green trail winds through the woods 3.7 miles. At this point on the blue trail, the surface becomes asphalt and you are heading toward the boathouse and recreational amenities, which include a food concession, bathrooms, a playground, picnic tables, and grills. Follow the trail and turn right at the southern end of the lake to cross over the dam and return to the nature center parking lot.

Cosca Regional Park

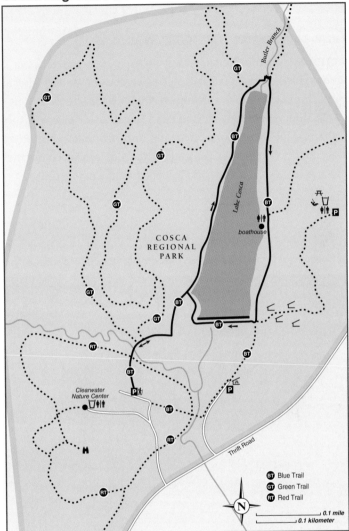

NEARBY/RELATED ACTIVITIES

Explore the Clearwater Nature Center, which houses exhibits and various living creatures, including Tumbleweed, a black-tailed prairie dog. Outside, visit the herb garden and the caged hawks, owls, and eagle guarding it (they're maimed birds that couldn't survive in the wild).

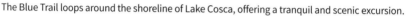

GPS TRAILHEAD COORDINATES N38° 44.031' W76° 55.055'

DIRECTIONS From the Capital Beltway (I-495) in Maryland, take Exit 7 and drive south on Branch Avenue (MD 5), heading toward Waldorf. After about 3.5 miles, turn right onto the 0.4-mile exit ramp leading to Woodyard Road (MD 223). Turn right onto Woodyard Road South. Go 0.8 mile, and turn left onto Brandywine Road. Go 0.9 mile and turn right onto Thrift Road. Go 2 miles and turn right at the Clearwater Nature Center sign. Follow the park entrance road 0.2 mile to the parking lot nearest the nature center.

The Blue Trail loops around the shoreline of Lake Cosca, offering a tranquil and scenic excursion.

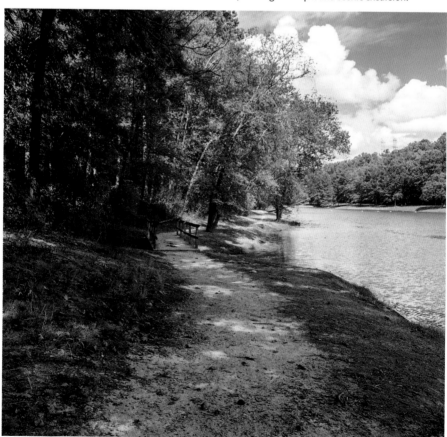

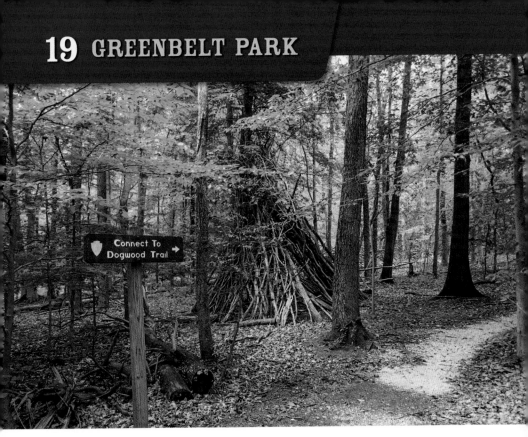

The Dogwood Trail offers extensive woodlands to explore.

SECRETED IN PRINCE GEORGE'S COUNTY, well-wooded Greenbelt Park is a great place to get fresh air and exercise, take in seasonal color, walk with friends, and contemplate life.

DESCRIPTION

Located a dozen miles northeast of the White House, Greenbelt Park ranks as the second-largest nature preserve within the Capital Beltway (after Rock Creek Park). Covering 1,100 acres, it is nestled amid a grid of major highways and suburban streets. Most of it remains undeveloped, with picnic areas and a campground being its major attractions. But it's also an attractive—if little-used—hiking locale. This hike is an easy 6.7-mile loop through the woods, with little elevation change. Each season offers an array of phenomena to observe. Only in a few places does the outside world intrude, and that's mostly in the form of traffic noise near the park boundaries.

The park is not a wilderness that has thwarted developers. Rather, it originated from an ambitious federal attempt at large-scale social engineering in the 1930s. Inspired by the international "garden city" movement, the Roosevelt administration bought up marginal and abandoned tobacco fields in Prince George's County.

LENGTH 6.7 miles (with shorter and longer options)

CONFIGURATION Modified loop

DIFFICULTY Easy

SCENERY Woodlands, stream valleys

EXPOSURE Lots of shade; less in winter

TRAFFIC Usually very light–light; heavier on weekends and holidays

TRAIL SURFACE Hard-packed dirt and sand; boardwalk and bridges in wet places

HIKING TIME 3 hours

DRIVING DISTANCE 12 miles

SEASON Year-round

ACCESS No restrictions

WHEELCHAIR TRAVERSABLE No

MAPS National Park Service, tinyurl.com/greenbeltparkmap; sketch map in free park brochure

FACILITIES Restrooms and water near Sweetgum picnic area near park entrance

CONTACT Park's on-site headquarters office, 301-344-3948, nps.gov/gree

LOCATION Greenbelt, Maryland

COMMENTS The park is Metro accessible—the hiking trail connects just over a mile from the College Park station (3 miles to the park entrance). It is very close to the Baltimore–Washington Parkway (I-295), so road noise is loud in some parts of the park.

It planned to create an experimental community shielded from Washington by a greenbelt of open land. But the plan was modified. The city of Greenbelt was duly built. Most of the open space, though, was incorporated into a sprawling United States Department of Agriculture research center. That left Greenbelt Park—formally taken over by the National Park Service in 1950—as the chief buffer zone. Over six-plus decades, the hemmed-in but well-protected tract has gradually evolved into a thriving woodland area that is rich in plant life. It also serves as a haven for such four-footers as deer, foxes, and groundhogs, as well as scores of bird species.

The hike begins at the main parking lot in the center of the park, just off of Park Central Road. Start at the trailhead for the Dogwood Trail on the west side of the parking lot. This is a short loop that connects the main road to the Perimeter Trail that runs around the edge of the park. At the first fork, you can walk either direction to get to the Perimeter Trail. You will come to a sign that says the longer route is to the left and the shorter route is to the right. They both loop to the same place, but we picked the left fork (longer loop).

Stay left until you reach a bench on the left side with an unmarked dirt trail behind it. Follow the dirt trail down a short incline to where it joins the Perimeter Trail, and turn right. Follow the yellow blazes clockwise around the park. (The park's major trails are color coded and well marked). Keep walking straight, cross a bridge, and bear left to stay on the trail; then turn right. This northern leg of the hike is a 2-mile segment that curves past a residential area and turns east, roughly parallel to the park's northernmost boundary. There it intersects the entrance road. Cross carefully, and then swing past the Holly and Laurel picnic areas. After

Greenbelt Park

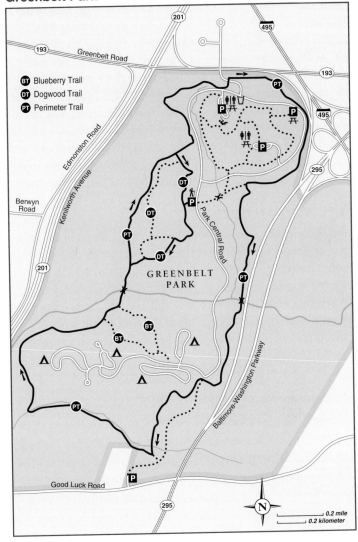

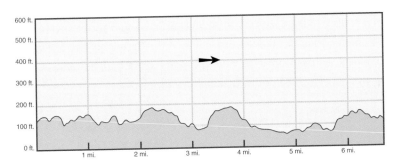

that, continue south, cross Still Creek, and hike roughly parallel to the Baltimore–Washington Parkway. Eventually the trail curves right and away from the parkway.

Head south to a boardwalk spanning a marshy area along a shallow stream called Deep Creek. At the next intersection, as you approach the campgrounds, you will see a sign that says TO METRO. Turn right and follow the Perimeter Trail left and then right, north, close to the park's western flanks. Anytime you reach an intersection, take the yellow-blazed option. After crossing a fire road and passing two side trails on the right (the second of which is the Blueberry Trail), you'll cross another stream, Still Creek (which lives up to its name about as much as Deep Creek does). At the final leg of the hike, turn right on the Dogwood Trail, and retrace your steps to the Dogwood parking area, or take the opposite loop to finish the hike in the other direction.

NEARBY/RELATED ACTIVITIES

Attend some of the park's annual events, held in the fall and in the spring on Earth Day. Explore the nearby city of Greenbelt and see what's left of the 1930s experimental community, including the Greenbelt Museum, 301-474-1936, housed in one of the community's original buildings on Crescent Road. Visit the nearby College Park Aviation Museum to see displays of aircraft and exhibits that tell the history of flight from the Wright Brothers to today, or stop at the NASA Goddard Visitor Center and check out the interactive exhibits describing space exploration programs.

• •

GPS TRAILHEAD COORDINATES N38° 59.305' W76° 53.832'

DIRECTIONS From the Capital Beltway (I-495) and I-95 in Maryland, take Exit 23 and head south 0.5 mile on Kenilworth Avenue (MD 201). Turn left onto Greenbelt Road (MD 193), head east for about 0.3 mile, and turn right into the park. Alternatively, from the Baltimore–Washington Parkway, head west on Greenbelt Road about 1 mile, and turn left into the park. Within the park, follow the winding entrance road 200 yards; turn right onto Park Central Road.

By Metro: Take the Green line to the College Park station. Walk east on Paint Branch Parkway. You will pass Corporal Frank Scott Drive and the Herbert Wells Ice Rink. Cross MD 201 (Kenilworth Avenue) and connect with the Perimeter Trail. Or take the Green line to the Greenbelt Metro station and connect with Metrobus C2; walk 100 yards to the park entrance. Contact Metro, 202-637-7000, wmata.com.

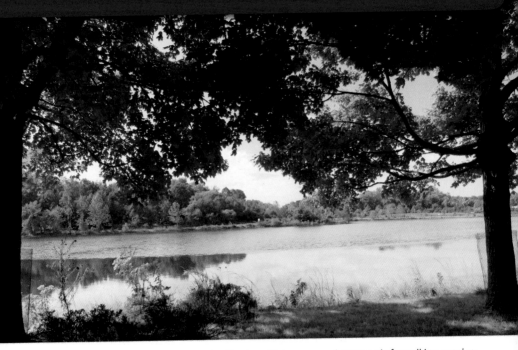

The paved trail surrounding Lake Artemesia offers beautiful scenery and easy terrain for walking, running, or bicycling.

THIS FLAT HIKE is a refreshing excursion through suburban Maryland just northeast of Washington. It features landscaped parklands, a man-made lake, and a streamside trail. The trail that encircles the lake connects to the hiker-biker Northeast Branch Trail and can easily be modified to extend the distance. This hike encompasses two loops to walk the full perimeter of the lake.

DESCRIPTION

Lake Artemesia, located in Prince George's County near College Park, consists of a 38-acre lake, a handicapped-accessible fishing pier, aquatic gardens, and several gazebos. Opened in 1992, Lake Artemesia Natural Area (named for Artemesia N. Drefs, a local resident) was created to repair damage to the natural landscape during the construction of the Washington Metro Green line. The lake has a healthy wild-life population, including deer, beavers, amphibians, and (during warm weather) too many bugs. The area is also popular with humans, especially on warm-weather weekends and holidays. Its paved trails are part of an evolving multiuse trail network known as the Anacostia Tributary Trail System.

LENGTH 3.8 miles (with longer and shorter options)

CONFIGURATION Modified loop and out-and-back

DIFFICULTY Easy

SCENERY Parklands, water views

EXPOSURE Mostly open; more so in winter

TRAFFIC Moderate; heavier on warm-weather weekends and holidays

TRAIL SURFACE Pavement

HIKING TIME 1.5–2 hours

DRIVING DISTANCE 12.5 miles

SEASON Year-round

ACCESS Open daily during daylight hours

WHEELCHAIR TRAVERSABLE Yes

MAPS USGS *Washington East*

FACILITIES Restrooms, water, and phone at lakeside building

CONTACT Prince George's County Department of Parks and Recreation, 301-627-7755, pgparks.com

LOCATION College Park, Maryland

COMMENTS Watch out for bicyclists, as this is a popular trail for them. The hike is Metro accessible, with the College Park station located just 0.7 mile from the trailhead. There is no on-site parking. Visitors can park south of the lake at the College Park Trail parking lot or the Calvert Road Park, and north of the lake at the intersection of 55th Avenue and Berwyn Road.

Lake Artemesia is a great place for fishing. The Maryland Department of Natural Resources stocks the lake with rainbow trout each year as part of the statewide Put-and-Take program. A nontidal fishing license is required for persons ages 16 and older. Warm weather brings color to the lake in the form of blossoming irises and water lilies. When the wind kicks up in the fall, the willows sway and you can hear the lake water lapping with relaxing low sounds by the shore. In winter, a glaze of lake ice and a dusting of snow can eerily bleach the scenery.

Begin the hike from the College Park Trail parking lot. Take the trailhead toward the woods, turning left at the first intersection and following the trail alongside a chain-link fence. You will pass the runway for the College Park airport on your left. If you are lucky you may watch a small plane take off or land. Walk over the footbridge, crossing the intersection with the Northeast Branch Trail, and continue straight ahead. Turn left through an opening in the fence, and turn left again on the lake loop trail. Follow the trail clockwise around the lake. As the water ends, turn right and then right again to follow the trail close to the water's edge. After passing the lake facilities, walk over the floating fishing pier to get a glimpse of the water. Then continue following the shoreline. As you complete this first loop around the southern section of the lake, cross the bridge and look for turtles paddling in the shallow water. Turn left on the trail to continue around the larger section of the lake. When you return to the lake facilities, take the trail left and stop to read the Wayside signs that describe the waterfowl and history of the lake. As you continue along the Lake Artemesia Trail, you may see great blue herons, Canada geese, mallards, wood ducks, or double-crested cormorants. When you reach the end of the trail, turn left

Lake Artemesia Natural Area and Northeast Branch Trail

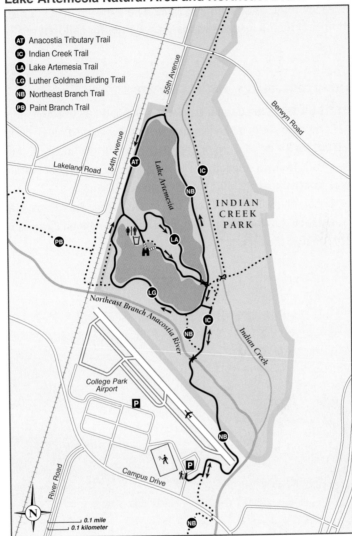

AT Anacostia Tributary Trail
IC Indian Creek Trail
LA Lake Artemesia Trail
LG Luther Goldman Birding Trail
NB Northeast Branch Trail
PB Paint Branch Trail

to recross the bridge. Then turn right, then left, and then right again to retrace your steps 0.8 mile along the Northeast Branch Trail back to the parking lot.

NEARBY/RELATED ACTIVITIES

Tour the College Park Aviation Museum (301-864-6029, collegeparkaviation museum.com), located on the grounds of the world's oldest continuously operating airport, which began in 1909 as the Army Signal Corps's first pilot-training facility under the tutelage of Wilbur Wright. The museum displays historical and reproduction aircraft and features hands-on activities for children of all ages.

• •

GPS TRAILHEAD COORDINATES N38° 58.611' W76° 55.269'

DIRECTIONS From the Capital Beltway (I-495) and I-95 in Maryland, take Exit 23 and head south 0.5 mile on Kenilworth Avenue (MD 201). Continue on MD 201 for 2.7 miles. Turn right onto Campus Drive. Turn right into the College Park Trail parking lot. The lot is located at the end of the airport runway adjacent to the Junior Tennis Champions Center.

Or use Metro: Take the Green line to the College Park Metro Station. Exit the station, turning left on River Road and then right on Campus Drive. Walk 0.5 mile to the parking lot and trailhead on the left.

Lake Artemesia is a scenic destination perfect for a leisurely stroll.

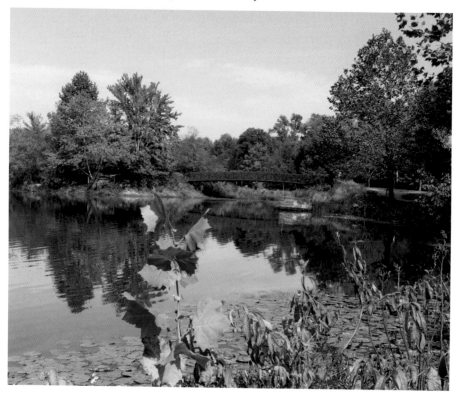

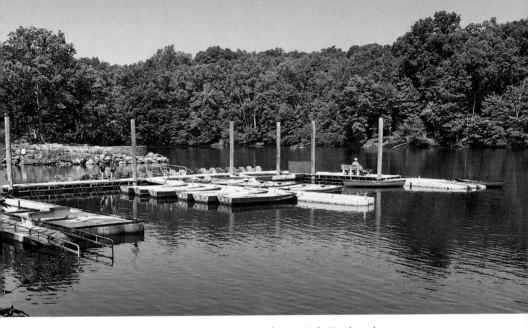

Along with hiking, fishing, and zip-lining, you can rent boats at Lake Needwood.

LAKE NEEDWOOD TRAILS consist of woods and open fields with near-constant views of the man-made, recreational lake fed by Washington's Rock Creek. This popular park offers a scenic shoreline trail in protected parkland nestled in the heart of suburban Maryland.

DESCRIPTION

At the turn of the 20th century, Congress recognized that the nature preserve built around Rock Creek was threatened by development upstream. They established a regional park system, Maryland–National Capital Parks and Planning Commission, in 1902 to protect a swath of land around the river called Rock Creek Parkway. Development continued in the region, until concerned citizens, led by Bernard Frank, organized the Rock Creek Watershed Association. In conjunction with the Wilderness Society, local citizens helped pass legislation that would protect the land and promote construction of two lakes using dams. One lake was named after Frank. In 1964, the ecologically minded residents passed zoning to inhibit urban overdevelopment with a program called Wedges and Corridors. The program was designed to save open space in stream valleys in the upper Rock Creek watershed.

LENGTH 2.5 miles

CONFIGURATION Loop around Lake Needwood

DIFFICULTY Easy

SCENERY Parklands, water views, boat dock and rentals

EXPOSURE Shady trails

TRAFFIC Light in winter; medium–heavy on warm-weather weekends and holidays

TRAIL SURFACE Gravel, mulch, and dirt

HIKING TIME 1.5 hours

DRIVING DISTANCE 30 miles (50 minutes with no traffic)

SEASON Year-round

ACCESS Open daily, sunrise–sunset

WHEELCHAIR TRAVERSABLE There are some paved trails around Lake Needwood.

MAPS Montgomery Parks, montgomery parks.org

FACILITIES Boathouse and snack bar with restrooms and water; boat rentals at lakeside building; hiker/biker trails; three picnic shelters; volleyball court; archery range; and Needwood Mansion (private facility).

LOCATION Rockville, Maryland

CONTACT Lake Needwood boathouse, 301-563-7540; Montgomery County Department of Parks and Recreation, 301-670-8080, montgomeryparks.org

In addition to providing water-quality control, the lakes have become a protected aquatic habitat while providing multiple recreational activities.

Lake Needwood is a 75-acre lake surrounded by parkland where visitors can rent rowboats, canoes, and paddleboats. The covered pavilion and snack bar also rents pontoon boats and picnic areas. People also come here to fish (you need a license) or play golf. The Rock Creek Hiker/Biker Trail begins at Lake Needwood and extends 14.5 miles into Washington, D.C. Go Ape Treetop Adventure has a few climbing platforms and zip lines (for ages 10 and older) built within the park. You are likely to see geese, chipmunks, squirrels, and deer.

Enter the park from Avery Road or Needwood Road, and follow signs for the boathouse on the southeast side of the lake. The Westside trailhead is found by the second of the two lots. Westside Trail starts out as a gravel path with a clear view of the lake on the right and an open field on the left. The path goes over the dam and then heads into a forest. On the right side of the path, you'll pass the remnants of a crumbling stone fireplace. You will pass two trails to higher ground—Parilla Path and Gude Trail, but continue to hug the shoreline on the Westside Trail and enjoy the clearings, where you'll get a panoramic view of the lake.

The trail goes uphill until you pass a pump house, where you will come upon the intersection of the Westside and Blue Heron Trails. Take the Blue Heron Trail to the left. The 0.78-mile trail climbs along the ridge until you get to Needwood Road. Turn right, and walk down the steps to walk along busy Needwood Road toward the Needwood Road entrance to the park. Cross the concrete bridge over the lake, and then turn right onto Beach Drive for a few feet until you see the Mudcat Trail heading into

Lake Needwood and Maryland's Rock Creek Regional Park

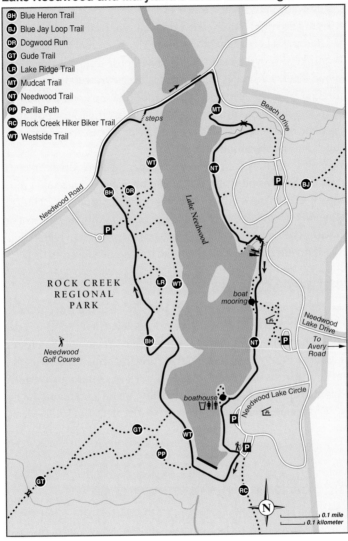

- **BH** Blue Heron Trail
- **BJ** Blue Jay Loop Trail
- **DR** Dogwood Run
- **GT** Gude Trail
- **LR** Lake Ridge Trail
- **MT** Mudcat Trail
- **NT** Needwood Trail
- **PP** Parilla Path
- **RC** Rock Creek Hiker Biker Trail
- **WT** Westside Trail

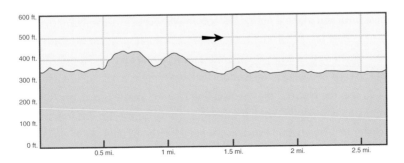

the woods. Follow the aptly named trail 0.18 mile along the shoreline until it intersects Needwood Trail. Turn right onto Needwood Trail, and continue through a picturesque marshy area. Be careful here as there are lots of roots and rocks on this path, but you'll enjoy the beautiful view of the island and the boathouse from this vantage point.

Needwood Trail, 1.15 miles long, crosses over two wooden bridges as it parallels the shoreline. You will also pass a boat mooring area and a swamp. When you come to the fork in the road, turn right again to stay by the lake. Continue past Picnic Area 2 toward the boathouse. After the boathouse you can access your car, but don't forget to check out the charming bear statue.

For a more vigorous and lengthy hike, consider the Rock Creek Hiker/Biker Trail, which starts at the Needwood visitor center and travels 14.5 miles south through Montgomery County's Rock Creek Stream Valley into Washington, D.C. The asphalt trail is made up of gentle hills and flat surfaces and has natural stopping points. The first is the crossing at Norbeck Road, at 2 miles, while a longer option is to hike 4.5 miles to Viers Mill Road. Visit tinyurl.com/rchikerbikermap to see a detailed trail map.

NEARBY/RELATED ACTIVITIES

Within Lake Needwood is the Go Ape Zip Line and Treetop Adventure Park (goape .com). Rockville Ice Arena (301-315-5650, rockvilleicearena.com) is located 2 miles from the lake. There are other hiking trails at Lake Frank, and youngsters will love Meadowside Nature Center (301-258-4030, tinyurl.com/meadowsidenature), with its live animals and birds of prey on display, as well as an indoor cave and slide. Lake Needwood is also about 5 miles from Rockville Town Center, with its huge library, art gallery, restaurants, shops, and grocery stores. The Rockville Metro station is close by.

• •

GPS TRAILHEAD COORDINATES N39° 06.887' W77° 07.690'

DIRECTIONS From the Capital Beltway (I-495) in Maryland, take I-270 North. Take the Montrose Road exit and keep left at the fork; follow the signs for Tower Oaks Boulevard. Turn left onto Tower Oaks Boulevard, and then travel 0.6 mile until you make a right on Wootton Parkway. Go 1.3 miles and continue onto First Street, which becomes Norbeck Road for 1.5 miles. Turn left on Avery Road. Follow Avery Road 2 miles until you turn left into the entrance to Rock Creek Park at Lake Needwood. Follow the signs to the boathouse.

Or use the Metro: Take the Red line train to Shady Grove, and catch Metrobus 53 on Redland Road to the Intercounty Connector. Disembark at Muncaster Mill/Needwood Road, and walk 1.3 miles to the Lake Needwood visitor center. Contact Metro, 202-637-7000 or wmata.com.

McKee-Beshers Wildlife Management Area offers scenic views and opportunities to view wildlife.

WEDGED BETWEEN THE POTOMAC RIVER and River Road in western Montgomery County lies a little-known wildlife management area where careful hikers can roam a splendid expanse of bird-rich crop fields, wetlands, woodlands, and hedgerows.

DESCRIPTION

It's easy to overlook the state-owned McKee-Beshers Wildlife Management Area (WMA), located on the Potomac River floodplain roughly 15 miles northwest of Washington. It is a secluded, 2,200-acre expanse of former farmland managed as habitat for game species and other wildlife. In July and August, more than 40 acres of sunflowers are in full bloom. The vibrant flowers grow up to 10 feet tall, with large yellow petals that are drawn toward the sun. Seven fields of flowers are planted each year in rotating locations. The Maryland Department of Natural Resources posts a map (see link in box) that shows the locations of the planted fields. You can also see the locations on your smartphone on Google Maps when you are on-site.

Please note that you can easily get into grassy areas that are difficult to navigate, so it is best to stay on well-groomed terrain. This 5.1-mile hike samples the WMA's

LENGTH 5.1 miles (with shorter or longer options)

CONFIGURATION Loop

DIFFICULTY Easy

SCENERY Crop and fallow fields, hedgerows, woodlands, tree reservoirs, other wetlands, river views

EXPOSURE Mostly open

TRAFFIC Usually very light

TRAIL SURFACE Mostly gravel; some grass

HIKING TIME 3 hours

DRIVING DISTANCE 33 miles

SEASON Year-round

ACCESS Towpath open daily, sunrise–sunset; elsewhere, no restrictions (but see text)

WHEELCHAIR TRAVERSABLE Partially, but not recommended

MAPS Maryland Department of Natural Resources, maryland.gov (sunflower map details change each year)

FACILITIES Restroom at towpath campground

CONTACT Maryland Department of Natural Resources' Wildlife & Heritage Service, 877-620-8367, maryland.gov

LOCATION Poolesville, Maryland

COMMENTS Acres of sunflower fields attract photographers and gardeners during the summer months. The grass trails are not well maintained, and online maps may not show updated areas that are best for hiking. Stay on trails where you can see the grass has been cut. Be aware of hunters December–September and mid-April–mid-May (see text); don't park on the Kunzang Palyul Choling temple grounds, especially on weekends.

fields, woodlands, hedgerows, and adjoining areas. Because the fields rotate each year, it is possible that an appropriate trailhead may be relocated. You should look carefully at the map to plan your route as not all trails connect.

The WMA trails are unblazed and unsignposted. And remember that the WMA is seasonally popular with both vicious insects and hunters. Avoid the bugs by staying away after rain from May to October, or use protective clothing and insect repellent. Avoid the hunters by staying away when they're active (visit dnr.state.md.us/wildlife for details).

To get started from the roadside trailhead, you'll pass a yellow-bar-gated, unpaved road leading south into the WMA. Follow the trail straight ahead. Some WMA fields are used to grow corn, sorghum, and other crops for humans; sunflowers, millet, and other crops for wildlife; and native grasses to furnish habitat for wild turkeys and other ground-nesting birds.

The trail will eventually become grass, and the last 50 feet or so may be planted with corn. If so, just walk through it. You will come to a narrow dirt path through the woods. Proceed straight and you'll reach the Chesapeake & Ohio Canal National Historical Park and the Potomac River across from Van Deventer and Tenfoot Islands. Take a right and follow the tree-shrouded towpath; remember that it is also a bike path, so stay to the right and yield to bikes. You will pass towpath milepost 27 and the Horsepen Branch Hiker-Biker campsite, which has a portable toilet, water pump,

McKee-Beshers Wildlife Management Area

picnic table, grill, and fire pit. Continue on the towpath 1.1 miles until you see a road to the right. Turn right and walk through the parking lot to continue onto the gravel-surfaced Sycamore Landing Road. Follow Sycamore Landing 0.8 mile. Turn right on River Road, walk another 0.3 mile, and turn right on Hughes Road. Hughes Road turns slightly left and becomes Hunting Quarter Road. After you pass through a parking lot, the road becomes a gravel road and passes by the "greentree reservoirs," where the WMA has manipulated water levels to provide habitat for waterfowl, wading birds, and numerous reptiles and amphibians. Continue another 1.1 miles back to the trailhead.

NEARBY/RELATED ACTIVITIES

Combine this hike with a 2-mile hike in the Kunzang Palyul Choling Tibetan Buddhist temple's nearby Peace Park. It's a lovely, wooded, and gently hilly area dotted with small meditation gardens and two of the traditional sacred Buddhist structures known as stupas. Pick up a trail map at the temple, and visit its website (tara.org/locations/maryland). If you do the WMA hike on a Sunday, try the temple's inexpensive buffet lunch. Also explore the temple itself.

• •

GPS TRAILHEAD COORDINATES N39° 04.900' W77° 23.369'

DIRECTIONS From the Capital Beltway (I-495) in Bethesda, Maryland, take Exit 39 to River Road (MD 190) heading west. Proceed 11.8 miles to the T junction where MD 190 ends but River Road turns left. Continue on River Road 3 miles. Turn left on Hunting Quarter Road, and park in the second parking lot on the left.

During the summer months, the gorgeous 10-foot-tall sunflowers are in full bloom.

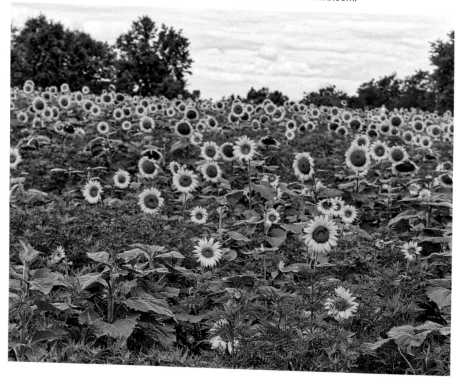

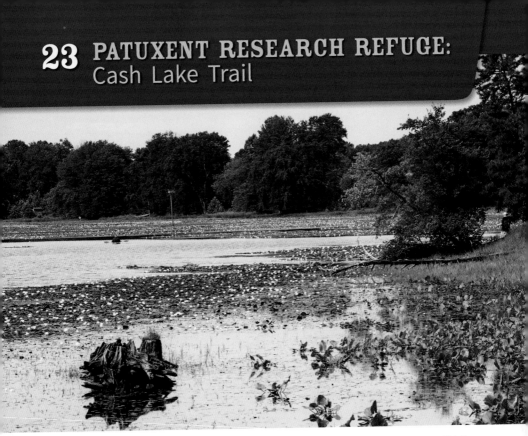

The hike encircling Cash Lake features picture-perfect scenery and the chance to see a variety of birds.

HIDDEN AWAY IN SUBURBAN MARYLAND between Washington and Baltimore lies a huge wildlife refuge where hikers can find a diverse and spacious landscape, open skies, many wild birds and animals, a few vestiges of the past, and much tranquility.

DESCRIPTION

As civilization relentlessly gobbles up open space between Washington and Baltimore, it's reassuring to know that 12,750 acres of land near Laurel remain—and will remain—gloriously undeveloped. Located mostly in Anne Arundel County (the rest is in Prince George's County), the acreage makes up Patuxent Research Refuge, which is run by the U.S. Fish and Wildlife Service as the nation's only national wildlife refuge devoted to wildlife and wildlife-habitat research. The refuge, which consists of deciduous and coniferous woodlands interspersed with wetlands and meadows, is a haven for myriad birds and land animals. It's also a safe and delightful place to enjoy solitude and tranquility while communing with nature.

The refuge was established in 1936 on mostly marginal farmlands and cutover woodlots bought up by the federal government for as little as $30 an acre. Subsequently

LENGTH 2.4 miles (with longer options)

CONFIGURATION Loop

DIFFICULTY Easy

SCENERY Woods, wetlands, meadows

EXPOSURE Mostly open; less so in months when sun is low in sky

TRAFFIC Generally very light; heavier on weekends and holidays

TRAIL SURFACE Dirt, gravel, boardwalks

HIKING TIME 1 hour

DRIVING DISTANCE 18 miles

SEASON Year-round, but a portion of the trail is closed seasonally to avoid disturbing wintering waterfowl. Best in spring and fall, especially for birders.

ACCESS The South Tract trails are open daily, sunrise–sunset. The National Wildlife Visitor Center is open daily (except Thursdays), 9 a.m.–4:30 p.m. The North Tract trails and visitor center are open daily, 8 a.m.–4 p.m. You must register to enter the North Tract

property. All trails and facilities are closed on federal holidays.

WHEELCHAIR TRAVERSABLE Partially

MAPS www.fws.gov/refuge/patuxent

FACILITIES Restrooms and water at visitor center, wheelchair-accessible restrooms at the Cash Fishing Area

CONTACT 301-497-5760; www.fws.gov/refuge /patuxent

LOCATION Laurel, Maryland

COMMENTS Patuxent Research Refuge offers many wildlife and habitat attractions. There are two areas of the refuge that are open to the public, the North and South Tracts. They are 10 miles apart. Although the brochures list many trails, most of them are paved roads that are better suited to bicycling and not ideal for hiking. The Cash Lake Trail and surrounding trails on the South Tract are the most scenic and best for wildlife viewing and photography. If you wish to visit the North Tract, hike the 2.5-mile Forest Trail, which offers a secluded walk through a hardwood forest.

more than quadrupled in size, the refuge now consists of three contiguous tracts. The open-to-the-public South Tract, which has an impressive visitor center and a few short and easy trails, attracts most of the refuge's human visitors. The closed-to-the-public Central Tract accounts for most of the research facilities. The open-to-the-public North Tract gets very few human visitors and has about 20 miles of trails that are mostly broad dirt-and-gravel or gravel roads. They're open to people on foot (including hunters, seasonally), as well as those on bikes, horses, and even skis.

The refuge is worth visiting at any time of year, but the greatest wildlife activity occurs in the spring and fall. More than 200 animal species have been recorded at the refuge, so we suggest taking along field glasses and a bird book (or an expert birder), plus the refuge's own bird checklist, available at the contact station. A wildflower book or an expert friend can also be seasonally helpful.

To get started on the hike, exit the door to the far left of the National Wildlife Visitor Center. Follow the trail and turn right to connect with the Cash Lake Trail. You will see a sign for Lake Redington on your right. Make an immediate left onto the boardwalk and follow it until you come to a wildlife-viewing blind, a great spot to look for birds. Take a right and follow the wetlands boardwalk, passing signs that tell you about the plants or birds you may see along the way, such as spatterdock, or

Patuxent Research Refuge: Cash Lake Trail

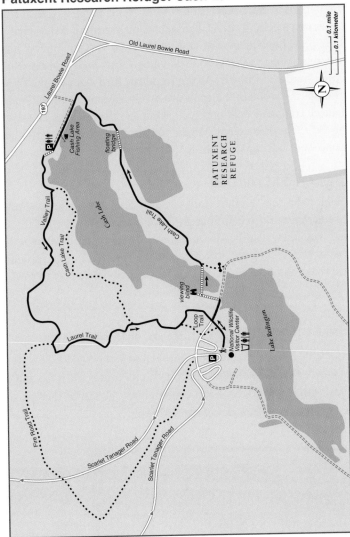

pond lily, a native perennial with shiny, heart-shaped leaves that can float on water, and the killdeer, a shorebird that is the size of a robin.

You will have a variety of views of the 53-acre Cash Lake as the trail winds in and out of the woods. Wildlife along the trail may include beavers, northern water snakes, fish, waterfowl, and songbirds. The terrain is varied but easy to navigate, ranging from gravel surface trails to boardwalks. You will even encounter a floating bridge with gorgeous white and pink water lilies floating in the lake (in summer). The trail is partially handicapped accessible (with access from MD 197/Laurel

115

Bowie Road) at the Cash Lake Fishing Area. Handicapped-accessible parking, a ramp that goes to a pier, and wheelchair-accessible restroom facilities are available.

Continue past the fishing area, and the trail narrows to a gravel footpath that enters the woods. Along the way, you will enjoy some shade and see features of the oak and beech hardwood forest. At the signpost, turn right onto Valley Trail and proceed through the woods. The trails are nicely groomed and well marked. Turn left onto Laurel Trail, and walk until you reach an opening in the woods. Continue straight toward the visitor center. When you come to an intersection, make a left onto the Loop Trail and continue straight to return to the visitor center.

NEARBY/RELATED ACTIVITIES

After the hike, take the Wildlife Conservation Tram Tour (301-497-5776, tinyurl .com/patuxenttramtours), a half-hour guided electric-tram tour that travels through forest, meadows, and wetlands. Also, take time to explore the exhibits at the National Wildlife Visitor Center, or participate in some of the refuge's public programs, which include bird walks and occasional evening hikes, including an Owl Prowl.

• •

GPS TRAILHEAD COORDINATES N39° 01.598' W76° 47.920'

> **DIRECTIONS** From the Baltimore–Washington Parkway (MD 295), take Exit 22 to Powder Mill Road/Beltsville. Go east on Powder Mill Road and drive 2 miles. Turn right into the visitor center entrance (Scarlet Tanager Loop). Go 1.4 miles to the visitor center parking area.

Aquatic plants and flowers float in the lake, making it a beautiful setting.

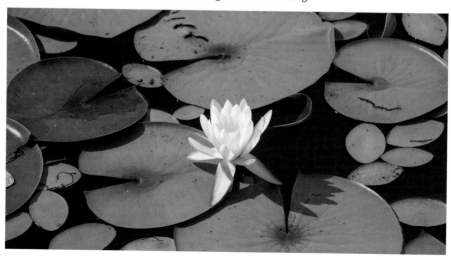

24 SANDY SPRING UNDERGROUND RAILROAD TRAIL: Woodlawn Manor Cultural Park

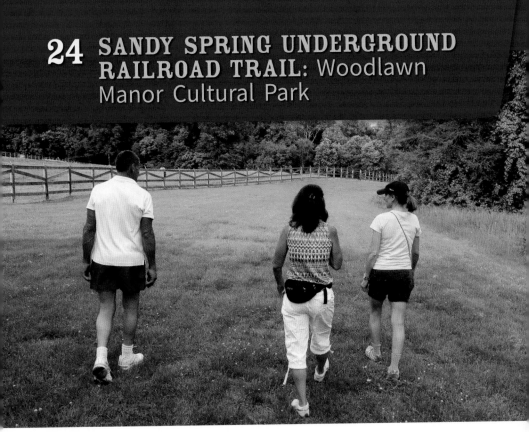

This grassy trail in suburban Maryland leads to Woodlawn Plantation.

THE SANDY SPRING Underground Railroad Trail, part of the National Park Service's Network to Freedom program, commemorates the involvement of Montgomery County residents in the Underground Railroad and celebrates the Quaker heritage and traditions of the Sandy Spring community. Hikers can follow the interpretive signs or join a guided hike with "conductors" who teach survival techniques used by escaping slaves. Guided hikes are offered April–November on Saturdays.

DESCRIPTION

In the 1850s, the Religious Society of Friends, or Quakers, had settled in this region, many becoming prosperous farmers. They worshipped at the Sandy Spring Meeting House and were morally opposed to slavery, having outlawed the owning of slaves in 1777. Here in Sandy Spring, many free blacks joined the community and were able to own their own homes and farms, as well as organize their own churches. Slavery had not yet been abolished nationally, so circulating in the community still remained extremely dangerous, even for free blacks, because of slave catchers who lurked in the woods.

LENGTH 4.2 miles (with shorter options)

CONFIGURATION Out-and-back

DIFFICULTY Moderate

SCENERY Woodlands, open fields, stream crossing, historic landmarks, horse pastures, plantation

EXPOSURE Mostly open, with some shade through the forest

TRAFFIC Usually light; heavier on warm-weather weekends; some guided tours

TRAIL SURFACE Dirt, gravel, road, rocks, roots

HIKING TIME 2 hours

DRIVING DISTANCE 29 miles

SEASON Year-round

ACCESS Open anytime

WHEELCHAIR TRAVERSABLE No

MAPS Montgomery Parks, montgomery parks.org

FACILITIES Restrooms at Woodlawn Manor Cultural Park's visitor center during open hours

CONTACT Montgomery County Park Headquarters, 301-495-2500, montgomeryparks .org; Woodlawn Manor Cultural Park (open April–November, Wednesday–Sunday, 10 a.m.–4 p.m.), 301-929-5989, montgomery parks.org/ppsd

LOCATION Sandy Spring, Maryland

COMMENTS The trail has some rough patches and is popular with dog walkers.

Sandy Spring's Quakers joined the free blacks to help escaping slaves make their way north. Landmarks on this trail include Sandy Spring and an impressive historic farm owned by the Maryland Park Service. The Woodlawn Manor Cultural Park is now used to demonstrate local history, host weddings, and provide interpretive hikes.

Start your hike by parking in the lot next to the Sandy Spring Meeting House. Walk along a paved road until you see the trailhead on a gravel path. Enter the trailhead via a gravel path with farms on either side, and walk until you come to an open pasture thick with grass and old-growth trees dating back to the 1700s.

At the fork in the road, pass through a yellow gate, and then turn left for a short detour to witness the majesty of a 300-year-old champion ash tree. Located at the edge of a suburban neighborhood, the tree was planted during the founding of the Village of Sandy Spring in the 1720s. The tree likely served as a landmark for people escaping on the Underground Railroad. Walk to the base of this ancient tree to read the sign that explains its history, and then return the way you came to reenter the Sandy Spring Trail on the gravel path.

The next landmark is the trail's namesake, the actual Sandy Spring, which is enclosed by a fence and covered by a concrete archway constructed in 1914. The date over the spring is when the Quakers held their first Friends meeting. The spring still provides a steady stream of cool water, the same water that sustained travelers on this trail for centuries and served as a trail marker for fugitives on the Underground Railroad.

The water feeds a creek that flows into the Northwest Branch of the Anacostia River. The sign outside the fence explains how the water is filtered by passing

Sandy Spring Underground Railroad Trail: Woodlawn Manor Cultural Park

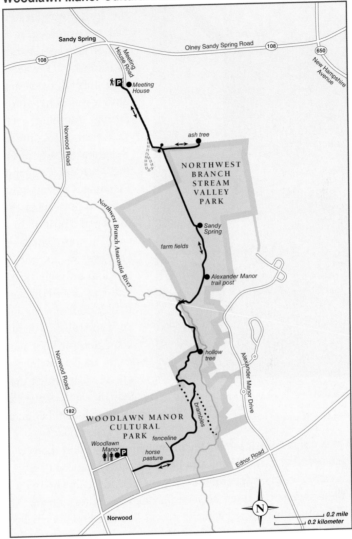

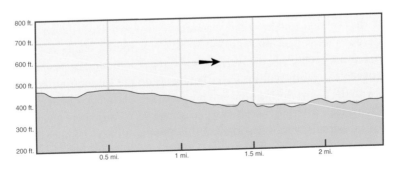

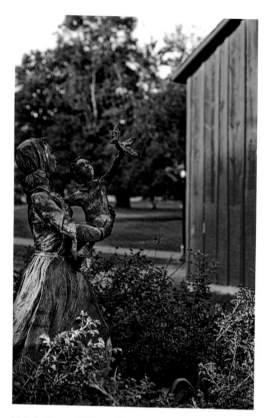

Visit the barn exhibits and learn about a bustling farm, its community, and those who made a bold bid for freedom on the Underground Railroad.

through the sandy soil. In 1745, the spring was located on what was once known as Snowdon's Manor and later became known as Harewood. Ownership of this land turned over many times, until it was donated to the Sandy Spring Museum, which now shares caretaking duties with the Religious Society of Friends and the National Capital Parks and Planning Commission, all dedicated to preserving the environment and "spirit of the spring."

The trail crosses a pasture—a very narrow dirt path with crevices and divots in the dirt. When fugitives passed through this way, they hid among the tall stalks of corn and tobacco plants. You may want to wear high socks or long pants to deal with the tall, wet grasses that crowd the tiny trail. Stay on the lookout for deer and other woodland animals crossing this grassy plateau.

You'll pass a sign for Alexander Manor neighborhood, and then enter a forest. There's a sign pointing to the Woodlawn Farm here directing you to cross a wooden bridge that is a replica of bridges built during the period leading up to the Civil War. Dogs and their owners can often be seen playing around this stream. Most escaping slaves did not know how to swim, so creeks like this posed a challenge. Sometimes a hidden boat would assist the slaves in crossing; otherwise, they depended on stepping-stones.

Follow the wooded trail up a hill, passing by an enormous Hollow Tree and Boundary Stone. Trees like this were often excellent hiding places for escaping slaves. It was also a good place to hide food or water. The Boundary Stone marked the line between two farms but was also a landmark on the Underground Railroad. Historians with the Sandy Spring Museum report that enslaved people seeking their freedom often escaped during the week of Christmas, when they were given time off and allowed to visit relatives or friends. Another popular time to escape was during a rainstorm, which helped wash away their tracks and kept dogs from following their scent. Forested areas like this provided excellent shelter and camouflage.

Another popular place to hide was the bramble patch, as the thorns deterred both animals and people. It's believed that fugitives chose this location to rest without worrying about being detected.

Continue through the forest, following the signs, until you come to a clearing and the elegant property known as Woodlawn Manor Cultural Park. Beautifully landscaped grounds surround the buildings here. The Federal-style brick house was built by a prominent Quaker family, who lived here between 1800 and 1815. The property has several champion trees, including a huge Osage orange tree with an 11-foot-diameter trunk. Don't miss the three-story stone barn converted into a visitor center with exhibits on Quaker heritage, African American communities, and the Underground Railroad.

There is a stable of horses, a gazebo, gardens, and a parking lot. Explore the grounds, and notice the statue of a young woman holding her child, who is reaching for a butterfly. It brings to mind the beauty and privilege of freedom. After you have had time to look around, return the way you came by heading back into the woods.

NEARBY/RELATED ACTIVITIES

Located on the grounds of the Sandy Spring Friends School is the Sandy Spring Adventure Park (240-389-4386, sandyspringadventurepark.org) with zip line adventures, a ropes course, and a labyrinth for younger kids. The small but fascinating Sandy Spring Museum (301-774-0022, sandyspringmuseum.org) has exhibits on cultural happenings in the community. The museum has a summer beer-and-wine garden and a year-round sculpture garden. Down the road, in nearby Olney, are multiple restaurants and shops.

• •

GPS TRAILHEAD COORDINATES N39° 08.855' W77° 01.543'

DIRECTIONS From the Capital Beltway (I-495), take I-270 North toward Frederick 8 miles. Take Exit 9A/9B to merge onto I-370 East at Sam Eig Highway toward the Shady Grove Metro Station. Continue 2.4 miles on I-370, which merges with MD 200 for 5 miles. Then take Exit 8B for MD 97 toward Olney. Continue 4.2 miles on MD 97/Georgia Avenue to MD 108 Olney/Sandy Spring Road in Ashton. Go east on MD 108, and make a right onto Meeting House Road to reach 17715 Meeting House Road, Sandy Spring.

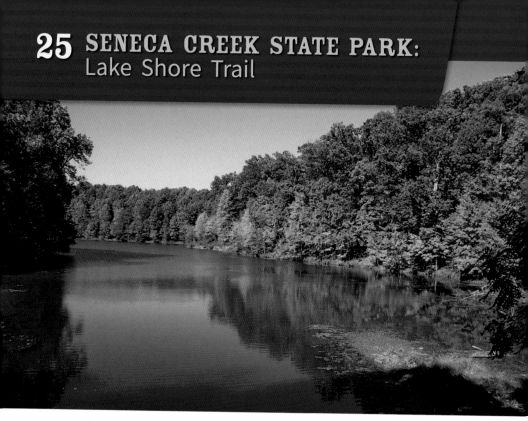

Clopper Lake at Seneca Creek State Park offers a beautiful destination for hiking, boating, and picnicking.

THE 3.6-MILE TRAIL loops around the 90-acre Clopper Lake at Seneca Creek State Park. The trail is well-maintained and offers one of the most scenic hikes in the area, with panoramic views of the lake all along the trail. It's a perfect outing for families.

DESCRIPTION

Seneca Creek State Park is a 6,300-acre, state-owned recreation area that offers facilities for boating and fishing as well as trails for hiking, cycling, and horseback riding. Clopper Lake was created for recreational use and flood control by damming Long Draught Creek, a tributary of Seneca Creek, in 1975. It is stocked with largemouth bass, tiger muskie, channel catfish, sunfish, bluegill, and pumpkinseed sunfish. The name Clopper has a rich history in the area, dating back to the 1800s, when Francis C. Clopper purchased more than 540 acres and an existing mill on Seneca Creek. The land remained in the Clopper family for four generations, until 1955, when the state purchased it to become part of Seneca Creek State Park. Throughout the park, there are traces of mill ruins and the Clopper home (near the visitor center).

LENGTH 3.6 miles

CONFIGURATION Loop

DIFFICULTY Easy

SCENERY Lake views, woodlands

EXPOSURE Mostly shady; less so in winter

TRAFFIC Usually light–very light; heavier on warm-weather weekends and holidays

TRAIL SURFACE Dirt

HIKING TIME 1.5 hours

DRIVING DISTANCE 30 miles

SEASON Year-round

ACCESS Open daily, 8 a.m.–sunset, March–October; 10 a.m.–sunset, November–February.

There is a $3/person day-use service charge on weekends and holidays, April–October; out-of-state residents, add $2.

WHEELCHAIR TRAVERSABLE No

MAPS Maryland Department of Natural Resources, maryland.gov

FACILITIES Restrooms at picnic areas

CONTACT 800-830-3974, maryland.gov

LOCATION Gaithersburg, Maryland

COMMENTS Mountain bikes are allowed on the trail. On the south side of the lake, you can follow the Mink Hollow Trail to connect to the Greenway Trail for a longer hike.

The Lake Shore Trail is well marked and easy to follow, with blue blazes on trees along the way. Begin the hike from the Chickadee parking lot (by the playground) or the Kingfisher Overlook parking lot that is at a vantage above the dam. You can walk the loop in either direction. The trail is shady with a wide variety of mature trees, including maples, oaks, pines, cedars, sycamores, and beeches. You will likely see ducks, geese, loons, blue herons, turtles, fish, and a variety of other birds. There is evidence of beavers in the area, as many of the trees have been cut by their powerful teeth. As you pass the boat center, look for the signs and blue blazes to stay on the trail.

More than 50 miles of trails are open for hiking, horseback riding, and bicycling in Seneca Creek State Park. The park also offers boat rentals, fishing, canoeing and kayaking, hunting, picnicking, playgrounds, a 27-hole disc golf course, and cross-country skiing. A tire playground is a local favorite for kids of all ages. Hunting is allowed in designated areas.

NEARBY/RELATED ACTIVITIES

The Woodlands, a short, self-guided trail located at the Clopper Day-Use Area park office, interprets the life and estate of the Clopper Family. Additional trails for hiking and biking nearby include the 16.5-mile Seneca Creek Greenway Trail (Hike 26, page 126) that follows the entire course of the creek and the 12-mile Schaeffer Farm Trail Area that is a favorite for mountain biking. For refreshments and a variety of homemade treats, stop at the nearby Lancaster County Dutch Market (lcdutch market.com; open Saturday, 9 a.m.–3 p.m., and closed on Sunday).

Seneca Creek State Park: Lake Shore Trail

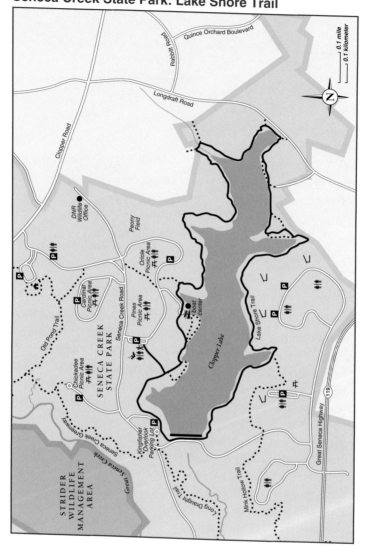

GPS TRAILHEAD COORDINATES N39° 08.742' W77° 15.172'

DIRECTIONS From Washington, D.C., Virginia, and points south, take I-270 north toward Frederick, Maryland. Take Exit 10 (Clopper Road/MD 117). Turn right at the light at the bottom of the ramp. The park is approximately 2 miles on the left.

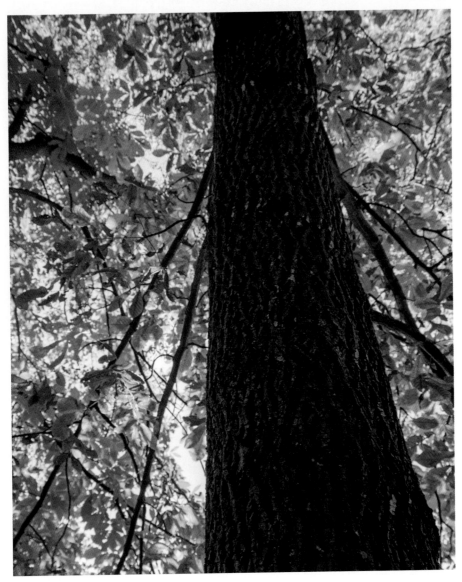

The trees surrounding Clopper Lake are especially beautiful when they change color in the fall.

From points north, take I-270 south toward Washington, D.C., and take Exit 11 (MD 124 West). Turn right at the light at the bottom of the ramp. At the second light, turn right onto Clopper Road (MD 117). The park is approximately 1.5 miles on the left.

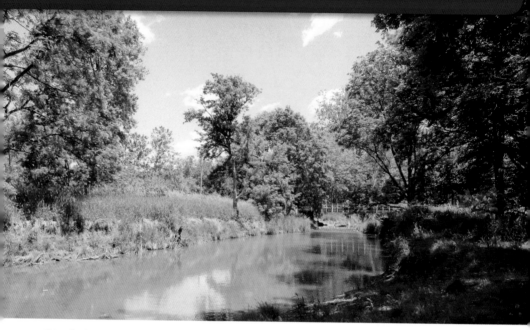

This suburban oasis offers a surprisingly quiet and wooded destination for hiking.

THE UNSPOILED AND LITTLE-USED Greenway Trail in Seneca Creek State Park features varying terrain and fauna along the pristine creekbed, making it one of the metro area's best close-in trails.

DESCRIPTION

Running the length of Seneca Creek State Park and beyond in west-central Montgomery County near Montgomery Village, the 25-mile-long Greenway Trail is one of the finest close-in hiking trails. It follows the creek from the Damascus area, where it connects with the Lower Magruder Trail (see Hike 47, page 217), down to the Potomac River at Riley's Lock (in Seneca), where it meets the C&O Canal Towpath. Officially called the Seneca Creek Greenway Trail, it was constructed over a decade-plus, mostly by a band of resolute volunteers who still plan to link the Damascus end with Patuxent River State Park. As of this writing, Seneca Creek Greenway is used for a trail marathon and 5K.

This out-and-back hike of 8.7 miles, with 900 feet of elevation change, uses a section of the trail located in Gaithersburg, about 25 miles northwest of Washington. It's a very scenic section, which mostly lies close to Great Seneca Creek, one of

LENGTH 8.7 miles (with shorter and longer options)

CONFIGURATION Out-and-back

DIFFICULTY Moderate

SCENERY Stream valley, woodlands

EXPOSURE Mostly shady; less so in winter

TRAFFIC Usually light; less so on warm-weather weekends and holidays

TRAIL SURFACE Hard-packed dirt; roots in places

HIKING TIME 3.5–4 hours

DRIVING DISTANCE 30 miles

SEASON Year-round

ACCESS Open daily, 8 a.m.–sunset

WHEELCHAIR TRAVERSABLE No

MAPS Montgomery Parks, montgomery parks.org

FACILITIES None

CONTACT Volunteers' website, senecatrail .org; Seneca Creek State Park, 301-924-2127

LOCATION Gaithersburg, Maryland

COMMENTS The trail is hilly and steep in sections and includes stream crossings. Watch for mountain bikers.

Seneca Creek's chief headwaters. You'll be in a serene and mostly pastoral landscape of wildflower-dappled floodplain areas, thickets, and wooded hills. Deer, smaller four-footed creatures, birds, wildflowers, and trees are plentiful. The trail is quite well blazed and signposted.

To get started from the MD 355 parking lot, take the trailhead to the right. The trail very quickly takes you from a highly trafficked road into a forest that winds up and down hills and over creeks, feeling like it is miles away from civilization. After crossing over a dike for sediment control and passing by the creek, the trail begins to steeply climb a hill. As you hike, listen for chattering kingfishers along the creek and the staccato calls of woodpeckers in the woods, and watch for beaver-felled trees. In muddy places, where deer tracks are common, look for the difference between males and females (female prints are more pointed).

When you reach Watkins Mill Road, exit the woods and turn right, walk along the sidewalk for a short distance, cross over the bridge, and carefully cross the road. The trail continues to the left and reenters the woods on the far side of the parking lot. Enjoy the varied terrain as you cross through a meadow with tall grass and then return to the woods again. When you reach Brink Road, turn around and walk back to your starting point. You can also begin the hike here and walk in the opposite direction.

NEARBY/RELATED ACTIVITIES

For a longer hike, explore or sample other sections of the Greenway, Lower Magruder Trail, or Clopper Lake Trail. Stop at Bruster's Real Ice Cream (240-631-1222, brusters.com) after your hike for some of the area's best ice cream, made daily.

Seneca Greenway Trail:
Frederick Road (MD 355) to Brink Road

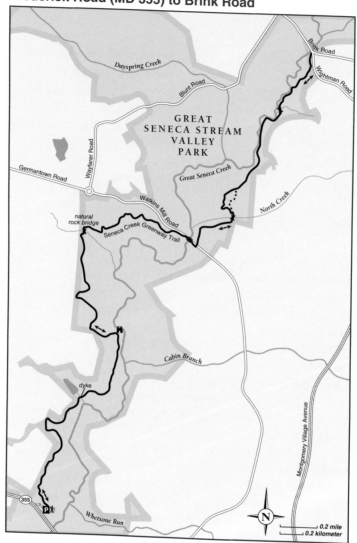

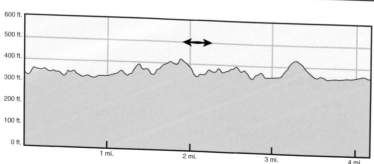

· ·

GPS TRAILHEAD COORDINATES N39° 10.042' W77° 13.739'

DIRECTIONS From the Capital Beltway (I-495), take I-270 North to Exit 11 (MD 124 North/Montgomery Village Avenue) in Gaithersburg. Take a left onto MD 355 North/Frederick Road. Follow MD 355 North 1.6 miles. The small parking lot and trailhead will be on the right shortly after you pass Game Preserve Road.

The trail runs along Seneca Creek with varying terrain, including woodlands and meadows.

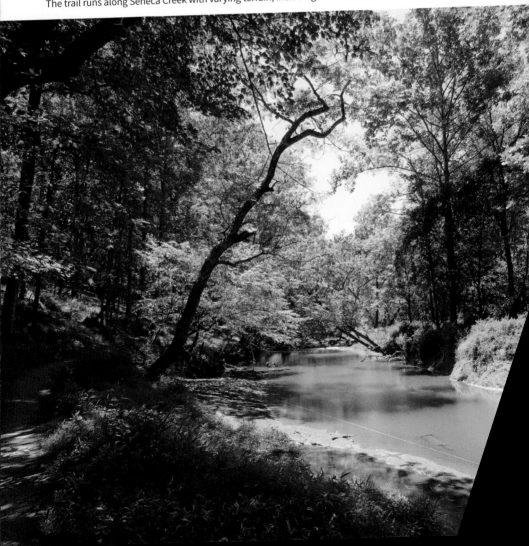

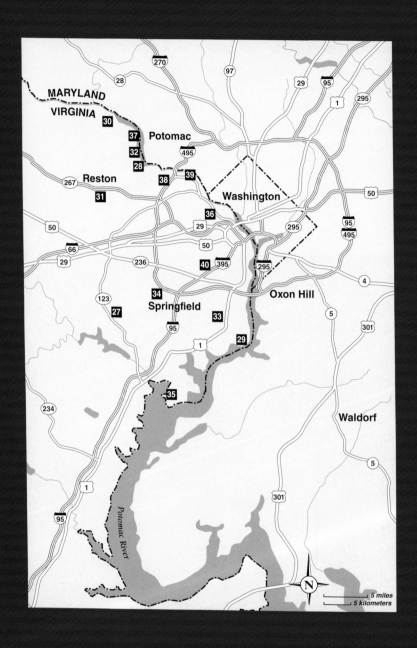

CLOSE-IN VIRGINIA SUBURBS (Alexandria, Arlington, and Fairfax Counties)

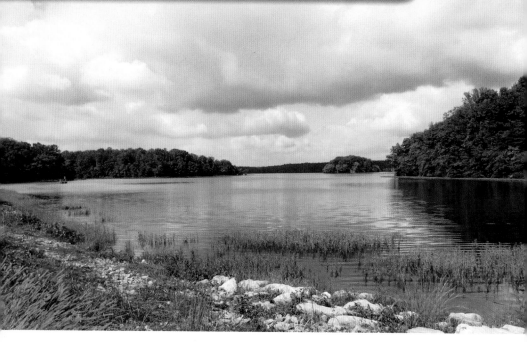

Burke Lake is a beautiful and popular site for walking, running, and picnicking.

THE 5-MILE TRAIL that loops around Burke Lake is well maintained and offers one of the most scenic hikes in the area, with panoramic views all along the trail.

DESCRIPTION

The 218-acre man-made lake was built on land in Fairfax County, Virginia, that was set aside by the federal government in the 1950s to build an airport. Protests from residents, as well as the rapid expansion of Washington's suburbs led to the construction of Dulles International Airport on its current site in Chantilly.

Burke Lake Park is operated by the Fairfax County Park Authority, while the lake is maintained by the Virginia Department of Game and Inland Fisheries. The lake is stocked with largemouth bass, muskie, crappie, channel catfish, bluegill, and walleye. Bald eagles and a variety of waterfowl can often be seen, including common, red-breasted, and hooded mergansers; common and red-throated loons; bufflehead, ruddy, and ring-necked ducks; and gadwall, pied-billed, and horned grebes. The loop trail traverses the lake and is well marked and easy to follow. It is very popular with local residents. You can begin from multiple locations and proceed in either direction.

LENGTH 5.1 miles

CONFIGURATION Loop

DIFFICULTY Easy

SCENERY Lake views, woodlands

EXPOSURE Mostly shady; less so in winter; short open stretch over the dam

TRAFFIC Moderate; heavier on warm-weather weekends and holidays

TRAIL SURFACE Dirt, gravel, and pavement on wheelchair-accessible segment

HIKING TIME 2.5 hours

DRIVING DISTANCE 25 miles

SEASON Year-round

ACCESS Open daily, sunrise–sunset; campgrounds open May–October. Day-use charges: weekends and holidays April–October, $10/per car; weekdays and November–March, no charge; free for Fairfax County residents.

WHEELCHAIR TRAVERSABLE Partially; access near boat ramp

MAPS Fairfax County Government, tinyurl.com /burkelakeparkmap

FACILITIES Restrooms at picnic areas, campgrounds, and boat ramp

CONTACT 703-323-6600

LOCATION Fairfax Station, Virginia

COMMENTS This is a popular destination for runners. Bicycles are allowed. Swimming and windsurfing are prohibited. State fishing license required for anglers over age 15.

Starting at the marina parking area and walking clockwise, you will soon pass the miniature train, the disc golf course, and the outdoor amphitheater. The Parcourse fitness trail begins on the west side of the lake and provides a circuit-training course with stations such as parallel bars, log hop, balance beam, body curls, sit-ups, and leg stretch. There are many benches along the perimeter of the lake that provide great vistas for photography and spots for resting.

On the west side of the lake, as you reach Burke Lake Road, follow the trail to the right and stay along the edge of the lake. From this point the trail passes multiple side access trails on the left as it continues around the lake. Stay on the main trail. On the east side of the lake, when the trail intersects with pavement, turn right to cross over the dam. This open section of the hike has one of the best views of the lake. As you continue, the trail becomes pavement (the south side of the lake near the boat-launch area) with wheelchair-accessible fishing platforms. Continue past the playground, cross the parking lot, and when you see a sign for the disc golf course, walk to the right to return to the marina parking lot.

NEARBY/RELATED ACTIVITIES

Burke Lake Park offers a variety of recreation opportunities, including fishing, boating, rowboat rental, camping, a miniature train, a carousel, outdoor volleyball courts, open fields, an 18-hole par 3 golf course, a driving range, disc golf, horseshoe pits, playgrounds, an amphitheater, and a minigolf course.

Burke Lake Park Trail

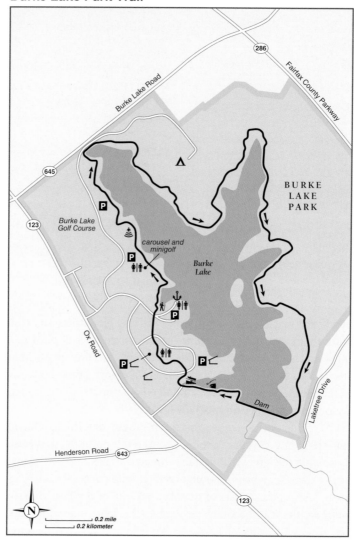

• •

GPS TRAILHEAD COORDINATES N38° 45.670' W77° 18.089'

DIRECTIONS From the Capital Beltway (I-495), take the Braddock Road West exit, and travel approximately 2 miles. Turn left onto Burke Lake Road (at Kings Park Shopping Center). Follow Burke Lake Road 5 miles. Turn left onto Ox Road (VA 123 South). The park entrance is the second left.

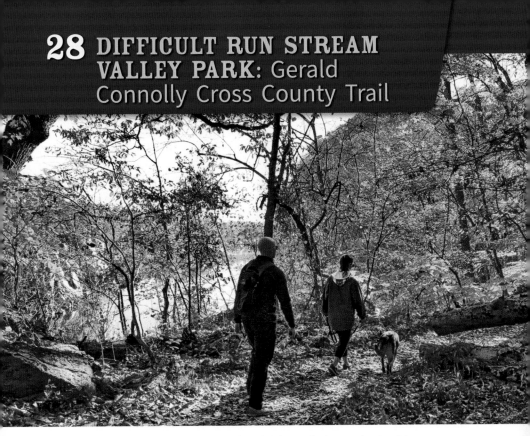

Difficult Run, at the southern edge of Great Falls Park, is known for its stunning riverside scenery.

DIFFICULT RUN STREAM VALLEY TRAIL follows the dramatic, fast-moving Difficult Run stream until it joins the Potomac River. The National Park Service maintains the well-marked trail with blazes and signage. Expect elevations over 300 feet with rocky, steep, and challenging sections of trail, plus extraordinary views of Mather Gorge, climbers scaling cliffs, and visitors exploring the riverbanks.

DESCRIPTION

Difficult Run stream is a 15.9-mile-long tributary that ends at the Potomac River's Great Falls Park. Populated by runners, hikers, dog walkers, and families, this relatively difficult trail (maybe that's how it got its name) was originally developed as a road used by the American Indians and later by colonists. The route was used to bring commerce from the Shenandoah Valley south to Georgetown. Centuries later, in 1974, the Old Georgetown Pike was paved.

The area is protected by the National Park Service and connects the Potomac Heritage Trail to the Gerald Connolly Cross County Trail (CCT), named in recognition of the Virginia congressman's efforts to establish more recreational sites for his

LENGTH 2.8 miles (with longer options)

CONFIGURATION Loop

DIFFICULTY Moderate–difficult

SCENERY Forested hills, rocky riverbank, cliff overlooks, rapids

EXPOSURE Shady; less so in winter

TRAFFIC Busy year-round; can be heavy on weekends and holidays

TRAIL SURFACE Dirt, rocky, boulder climbs

HIKING TIME 2 hours (with stops to watch climbers and explore riverbank)

DRIVING DISTANCE 19 miles

SEASON Year-round; lovely in winter

but best in fall and spring

ACCESS Open daily, sunrise–sunset

WHEELCHAIR TRAVERSABLE No

MAPS National Park Service, tinyurl.com /greatfallsmap

FACILITIES No restrooms or water, mostly wilderness hiking

CONTACT 703-757-3103, nps.gov/grfa

LOCATION Georgetown Pike, McLean, Virginia

COMMENTS This premier hiking trail is part of Great Falls Park and is overseen by the National Park Service. It is a small section of the 41-mile Gerald Connolly Cross County Trail. Dogs must be on a leash.

constituents. The CCT runs from the Potomac River to Occoquan Regional Park in southern Fairfax County.

Located between Scott's Run and Great Falls Park, the trailhead is at the edge of the gravel parking lot on Georgetown Pike/MD 193 and is marked with blue blazes. Difficult Run Trail parallels the stream, which cascades over enormous boulders with fast-moving rapids. The views are impressive, and it's hard to resist stopping frequently to admire such gorgeous cliff valleys.

The trail follows the stream for the entire leg down to the Potomac River. After 0.3 mile, it passes under the MD 193 bridge. Shortly after the bridge, you'll come to a sign marking the entrance to Great Falls Park with a map of hiking trails.

The Difficult Run watershed is the largest watershed in Fairfax County. It is home to 163 varieties of bird species, muskrat, beaver, ducks, geese, herons, and venomous copperhead snakes, so avoid any snakes you see hiding among the rocks. While we hiked early one morning, we saw a red fox bounding up the hill. Mature native trees, including sycamore, tulip, and beech, border the streambed. During a conservation effort in 1993, Fairfax County planted 1,019 native hardwood trees on this land.

The rapids and boulders become even more dramatic as the river creeps closer to the Potomac confluence. Continue straight on the Difficult Run Trail at the intersection with the Ridge Trail, and follow signs pointing you toward the Potomac River. Watch your footing, as this smooth gravel trail becomes rocky and steep. Make your way to the overlook, where you'll have a clear view of the confluence of Difficult Run and the Potomac River. After taking in the views, turn around and go back up the hill. This time, turn right at the Ridge Trail sign marker. At the top of the

Difficult Run Stream Valley Park: Gerald Connolly Cross County Trail

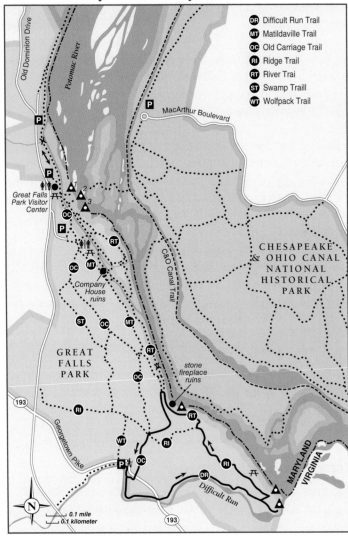

DR Difficult Run Trail
MT Matildaville Trail
OC Old Carriage Trail
RI Ridge Trail
RT River Trai
ST Swamp Traill
WT Wolfpack Trail

Old Dominion Drive

Potomac River

MacArthur Boulevard

Great Falls
Park Visitor
Center

C&O Canal Trail

CHESAPEAKE
& OHIO CANAL
NATIONAL
HISTORICAL
PARK

Company
House
ruins

GREAT
FALLS
PARK

stone
fireplace
ruins

193

Georgetown Pike

Difficult Run

MARYLAND
VIRGINIA

N

0.1 mile
0.1 kilometer

193

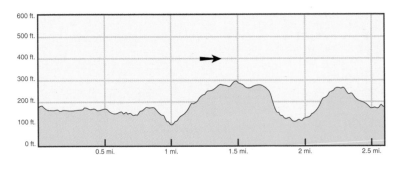

ascent, check out the second overlook on the right before turning left to continue on the Ridge Trail; follow the sign pointing toward Great Falls Park Visitor Center.

Soon you'll come to a picnic table on the right near a third Potomac River overlook called Cow Hoof Rock, a 30- to 50-foot-high crag. If you climb carefully out over Cow Hoof Rock, you may find rock-climbers scaling this steep cliff face. Turn right on the River Trail to descend wooden steps. Look across the river to see hikers on the rugged Billy Goat Trail in Maryland, and you may also see a few paddlers on the river below.

Keep looking for blue blazes, as the trail gets somewhat confusing after this. Rather than a gravel or dirt path, it proceeds by scrambling over deep crevices and large boulders. Shortly you'll come to the ruins of a stone and brick fireplace. Then, at the next fork, turn left on the Matildaville Trail, which makes a sharp, almost U-turn back up the hill. At the next trail marker, cross the Ridge Trail, and in 50 feet turn left on the much larger, wide-open Old Carriage Road Trail.

When you get to busy Georgetown Pike, cross carefully. This is a blind curve for drivers coming from the right, and most cars are going very fast. After crossing the road, turn right on the trail. At this point, you are retracing your steps on the Difficult Run Trail. When you enter the stream valley, continue on the trail as it jogs sharply right. You'll see the parking lot ahead of you.

NEARBY/RELATED ACTIVITIES

If you're up for more hiking or would like to try paddling, drive to Riverbend Park Visitor Center (Hike 37, page 174). To see the magnificent Great Falls, continue your hike toward the Great Falls Tavern Visitor Center (Hike 15, page 80).

• •

GPS TRAILHEAD COORDINATES N38° 58.698' W77° 14.938'

> **DIRECTIONS** From I-495, take Exit 44 for VA 193/Georgetown Pike. Go west onto VA 193 West/Georgetown Pike, following signs for Great Falls. After 3.6 miles, turn left into the Difficult Run parking lot, 8801 Georgetown Pike, McLean, VA.

29 FORT HUNT PARK AND MOUNT VERNON TRAIL

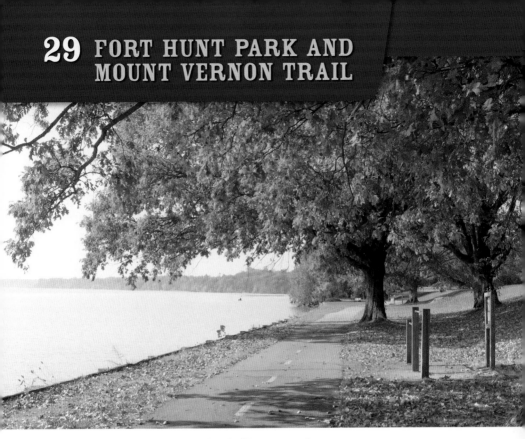

The scenery along the Potomac River is breathtaking year-round.

THIS HIKE STARTS WITH A LOOP through Fort Hunt Park and then leads to an out-and-back excursion on the Mount Vernon Trail, providing hikers with a lovely parkland outing along the Potomac River.

DESCRIPTION

In the 19th century, George Washington's former Mount Vernon estate became a de facto national shrine. Then, in the 1930s, the federal government created the scenic George Washington Memorial Parkway to carry motor vehicles down to Mount Vernon from Key Bridge, across from his namesake city. In 1973, it added the Mount Vernon Trail, a paved path in the parkway right-of-way for people who like to locomote by muscle power. Today, the 18-mile-long trail attracts hikers, bikers, runners, skaters, dog walkers, and strollers. It's officially part of the Potomac Heritage National Scenic Trail and serves as the core segment of this hike.

This 7.6-mile, mostly out-and-back, level hike uses the trail's lowermost portion. That's where the southbound Potomac River turns west and the Virginia riverbank becomes a picturesque corridor of open parklands, woods, and across-the-water views. The hike also includes part of Fort Hunt Park. Located on former

LENGTH 7.6 miles (with shorter and longer options)

CONFIGURATION Loop and out-and-back

DIFFICULTY Easy–moderate

SCENERY Parklands, woodlands, river views

EXPOSURE Mostly open

TRAFFIC Usually light; moderate–heavy on warm-weather evenings, weekends, and holidays

TRAIL SURFACE Pavement

HIKING TIME 3–3.5 hours

DRIVING DISTANCE 14 miles

SEASON Year-round

ACCESS Sunrise–sunset

WHEELCHAIR TRAVERSABLE Yes

MAPS National Park Service, tinyurl.com/mtvernontrailmap and tinyurl.com/fthuntparkmap

FACILITIES Restrooms and phones at Fort Hunt Park and at Mount Vernon (cafeteria too); portable toilets along trail

CONTACT George Washington Memorial Parkway office, 703-289-2500, nps.gov/gwmp

LOCATION Alexandria, Virginia

COMMENTS This is a busy hiker-biker trail; stay to the right and yield to bicycles. The trailside markers count down to Mount Vernon. There are several parking lots along the way, so you can easily shorten the hike by skipping the trek through Fort Hunt Park and parking closer to Mount Vernon. But note that the best views are closer to the 2-mile marker, where the trail is more open to the Potomac River.

Washington-owned land, the fort existed from the 1890s to about 1920 to guard the river approach to the capital. It was converted into a park in the 1930s.

To get started from the parking lot, head back toward the park entrance. But at the T junction, walk straight on the loop road, keeping right. Continue to walk clockwise around the loop road, traversing through most of the park past ballfields, picnic pavilions, and the United States Park Police substation and Fort Hunt Stables. The park loop road is lined with a variety of trees that have gorgeous color in the fall.

After passing the parking lot where you started, turn left at the T junction and head for the park entrance. En route, take an optional detour to look at an 1890s gun emplacement, on the right. Or visit another one, down a short trail just outside the entrance. Outside the park, carefully head downhill and cross a traffic intersection to reach the Mount Vernon Trail at an information board. Turn right and follow the trail. Stay left where it joins a roadway to curve through an underpass (that's the parkway above). Then turn right to rejoin the trail.

Proceed on the riverbank trail and savor the views. Watch for geese and ducks on the water, ospreys on the hunt, and bald eagles on the wing. Pause to look for the resident eagles nicknamed George and Martha (the names stay the same, but the birds occasionally get replaced by aggressors). At milepost 2, there are picnic tables and a parking lot. A Fit Trail begins here and proceeds along the route, with more than a dozen exercise stations. Continuing on the trail, you will pass boardwalks, swampland, the Cedar Knoll restaurant, and Riverside Park.

Fort Hunt Park and Mount Vernon Trail

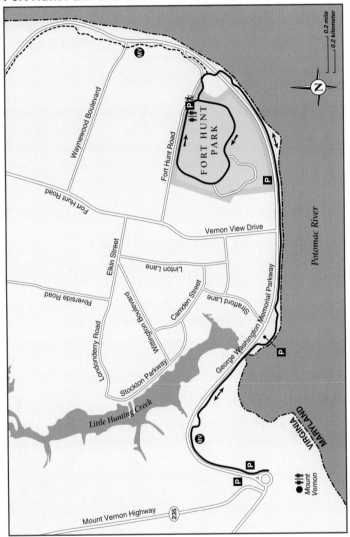

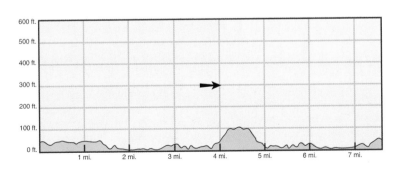

The trail leaves the shore and uses a long uphill slope to reach milepost 0 and the Mount Vernon parking lot. You cannot see much of the estate, as it is set back from the entrance. When you're ready, walk back the 3.4 miles to Fort Hunt Park.

NEARBY/RELATED ACTIVITIES

Visit the Mount Vernon Estate and Gardens (703-780-2000, mountvernon.org) to learn about the life of George Washington. The estate includes a 14-room mansion, outbuildings (kitchen, slave quarters, smokehouse, coach house, and stables), four gardens, and a museum and education center. In the summer, attend a Sunday-evening concert at Fort Hunt.

• •

GPS TRAILHEAD COORDINATES N38° 43.009' W77° 02.988'

DIRECTIONS From the Capital Beltway (I-495) in Alexandria, Virginia, take Exit 177B to get on northbound US 1. At the first traffic light, turn right onto Franklin Street, drive three blocks, and turn right onto South Washington Street, which becomes George Washington Memorial Parkway. At the city's southern end, proceed on the parkway 5.6 miles, and take the exit ramp to Fort Hunt Park. Enter the park, turn right onto the loop road at the T junction, and then take the first left, into the parking lot.

The trail features a mix of paved and boardwalk surfaces and is an easy place to walk, run, or bike.

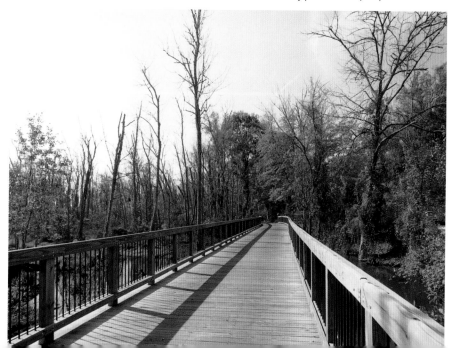

30 FRASER PRESERVE

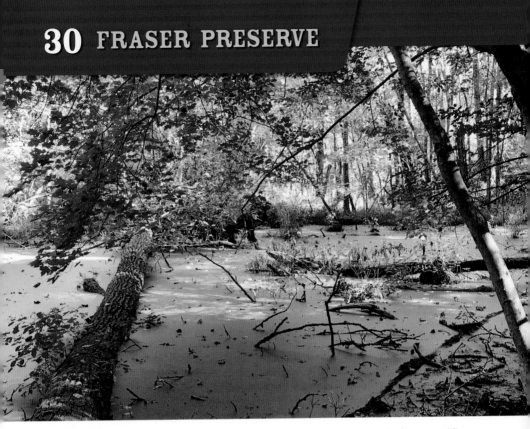

Along with the region's largest vernal pool, many different types of trees grow in the forest, providing a shady habitat for birds and animals.

FRASER PRESERVE IS A PRIVATE NATURE SANCTUARY in the northwestern corner of Fairfax County, close to the Potomac River. It's open to the public and is a delightful and secluded place to hike.

DESCRIPTION

Fraser Preserve is a 220-acre tract of rolling woodlands and floodplain some 14 miles northwest of Washington. Formerly a Washington family's summer refuge, the property was bequeathed to the Nature Conservancy in 1975 by Bernice Fraser. The land was once part of a tract of 5 million acres granted by King Charles I in 1649. The land passed through several hands, including Thomas Lee, one of the Virginia Lees. It was farmed until World War I, when Fairfax stopped functioning as a predominantly agrarian society. Fraser granted part of the land to Calvary Baptist Church, which joins the Nature Conservancy in protecting the preserve in its natural state for the enjoyment of visitors.

A small portion of Fraser Preserve is used as a children's camp with a climbing wall and screened-in porches. A single-lane paved road links the preserve's gated entrance to a cleared area containing the camp's lodge and a caretaker's cottage.

LENGTH 2.7 miles	**ACCESS** No restrictions
CONFIGURATION Balloon loop	**WHEELCHAIR TRAVERSABLE** No
DIFFICULTY Easy–moderate	**MAPS** Sketch map at kiosk; tinyurl.com
SCENERY Woodlands, camp, pool, wetlands	/fptrailmap. You can download an audio tour
EXPOSURE Mostly shady; less so in winter	map at tinyurl.com/fpaudiotourmap.
TRAFFIC Very light–light; occasionally heavier when camp is in session	**FACILITIES** No restrooms. Campground is not open to the public.
TRAIL SURFACE Dirt, gravel; rooty and steep in places	**CONTACT** National Conservancy, tinyurl.com /fraserpreserve; Northern Virginia Regional Park Authority, 703-273-0905, novaparks.com
HIKING TIME 1.5 hours	**LOCATION** Great Falls, Virginia
DRIVING DISTANCE 24 miles	**COMMENTS** Don't drive into preserve, even if
SEASON Year-round, sunrise–sunset	gate is open. Dogs are not permitted.

Yet most of the preserve is untamed woodland, in keeping with the conservancy's emphasis on eco-preservation. Mature deciduous trees dominate the hillsides, with a sprinkling of pines, hollies, and spicebushes providing wintertime color. During the warm-weather months, wildflowers flourish, and resident animals range from deer to salamanders. It is an especially good place to spot and hear local birds, including wild turkeys, sparrows, northern cardinals, and singing wood thrush.

This hike is a 2.7-mile balloon loop on reasonably well-maintained trails, with about 400 feet of elevation change. To get started, park in the gravel lot on Springvale Road. Walk through the gate on the gravel trail/road into the preserve (watch out for the occasional school bus or other vehicle that has permission to drive into the park).

Follow the narrow paved road that gently descends about 0.5 mile before crossing a concrete-and-stone bridge over a fast-moving stream named Jefferson Branch (in a few feet it becomes Nichols Run). Enjoy the dappled sunlight and gentle sounds of nature all around as your hike starts a slow uphill climb. Next you'll pass the camp houses, a fenced-in garden, and a driveway on your right before you come to the end of the road. Turn left onto the blue-blazed West Trail, but pause first at the kiosk to get your bearings.

This narrow dirt trail is flanked by bushes and a thick forest canopy. Continue on the West Trail as it opens up to a meadow. As you proceed to the bottom of a hill, you'll encounter a swamp forest with wetlands rich in diverse plants. In warmer weather, look for the deciduous bayberry bushes that give off a lovely scent. You'll also pass a stand of papaw trees—the fruit is an important food source for many animals, including swallowtail butterflies that lay eggs on the leaves.

Continue downhill and remain on the blue trail. There is a sewer line right-of-way that routes sewage to the water treatment plant, but you only notice it when

Fraser Preserve

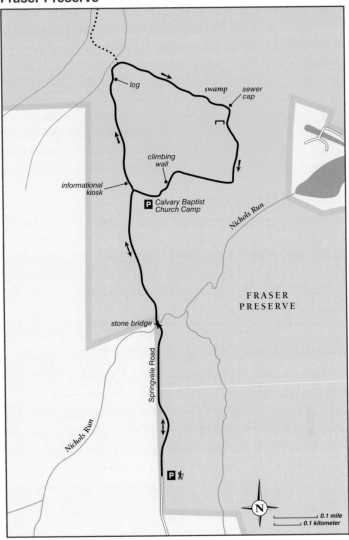

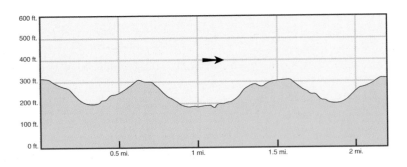

you see a sewer cap on the trail. Right after the cap, murky wetlands give way to the largest vernal pool in northern Virginia—a favorite habitat of the wood frog. Vernal pools are temporary, created by the seasonal rising and falling of the water table. In winter it's often covered with ice, and during the warmer months, with tiny duck-weed plants. Sometimes you can see turtles sunbathing on fallen tree trunks.

Stay on the blue trail as it passes a log bench, and then you'll come to a clearing. This area serves as a campground, with a screened-in porch and climbing wall. Camp Fraser is a living classroom sponsored by the Calvary Baptist Church in Washington. There are a few picnic tables around here. After passing the camp compound, the trail ends and you rejoin the gravel road, heading back to the parking lot.

NEARBY/RELATED ACTIVITIES

In addition to the Nature Trail, try hiking the River Trail. You will be on low bluffs bordering the Potomac River, which is visible through the trees. Just 15 minutes north, play a round of golf at the public Algonkian Golf Course (703-450-4655, novaparks.com/golf/algonkian-golf-course). Just 15 minutes south, visit Riverbend Park (Hike 37, page 174), where you can hike and paddle.

• •

GPS TRAILHEAD COORDINATES N39° 02.195' W77° 18.587'

DIRECTIONS From the Capital Beltway (I-495) in McLean, Virginia, take Exit 44 to get onto Georgetown Pike (VA 193) heading roughly west. Proceed 7.7 miles, passing through the community of Great Falls at the 6.3-mile mark. Then turn right at the traffic light onto Springvale Road (VA 674) and proceed 2 miles. Just after Beach Mill Road comes in from the right, fol-low Springvale as it makes a sharp left at the yellow arrow, continue about 25 yards, and take the first right to get back on Springvale (which cleverly becomes VA 755) to 239 Springvale Road.

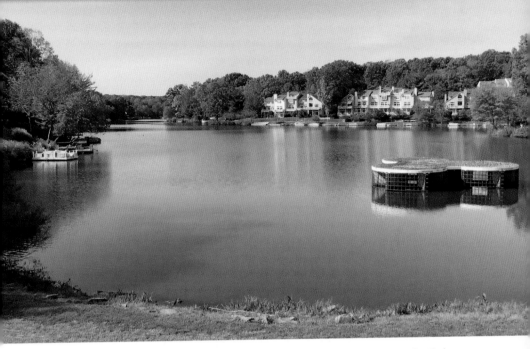

Hikers get a glimpse of Lake Audubon as they begin their trek through Glade Stream Valley Park.

THE TURQUOISE TRAIL is a 4.7-mile paved recreation trail in Glade Stream Valley Park that runs through Reston from South Lakes Village Center to Hunter Woods Village Center. The Reston Association Pedestrian and Bicycling Advisory Committee created the trail markings.

DESCRIPTION

Reston has five paved and natural-surface pathways winding 55 miles through its suburban neighborhoods. The Turquoise Trail is the longest of these trails and offers natural scenery as well as a connection to neighborhoods, recreation areas, and shopping centers. The trail provides an urban escape and is mostly flat and shady.

To access the trail, park at the Lake Audubon Pool (operated by the Reston Association). Enjoy a view of the lake, and then walk toward Twin Branches Road; turn right onto the sidewalk along the eastern edge of the lake. Pass by the Lake Audubon dam, continuing along the side of the road. Cross over Glade Drive and then enter the woods at the trailhead, where you will see a map for Glade Stream Valley Park. Here you're on a section of the Gerry Connolly Cross County Trail (CCT of Fairfax County, Virginia).

LENGTH 4.7 miles (with shorter options)

CONFIGURATION Out-and-back

DIFFICULTY Easy

SCENERY Stream views, woodlands, neighborhood

EXPOSURE Mostly shady; less so in winter

TRAFFIC Light; heavier on warm-weather weekends and holidays

TRAIL SURFACE Pavement

HIKING TIME 2.5 hours

DRIVING DISTANCE 24 miles

SEASON Year-round

ACCESS No restrictions

WHEELCHAIR TRAVERSABLE Yes

MAPS Reston Association, tinyurl.com /gsvptrailmap

FACILITIES Portable toilet at pool parking lot

CONTACT fairfaxcounty.gov, reston.org

LOCATION Reston, Virginia

COMMENTS This is a hiker-biker trail with lots of entrances and exits to surrounding neighborhoods. Expect to encounter walkers, joggers, bicyclists, wheelchair users, and pathway-maintenance vehicles.

Follow the paved trail. Shortly after the stream, turn right, following the Reston Association markers toward Hunter Woods. You are now on the Turquoise Trail. The trail goes past the wooded lots of beautiful homes to the right and follows a stream and meadow on the left. Turn right at the next intersection and stay on the trail for the rest of your hike. Be sure to enjoy the many scenic views along the way. Trees in the stream valleys include river birch, sweetgum, papaw, and species of willow and alder. On a quiet day, you may see wildlife such as birds, deer, muskrat, fox, and other critters. As this is an out-and-back hike, you can turn around at any point and retrace your steps back to your car.

The Gerald Connolly Cross County Trail, which passes through Glade Stream Valley Park, is a beautiful trail that extends through Fairfax County and is popular for a close-in neighborhood hike.

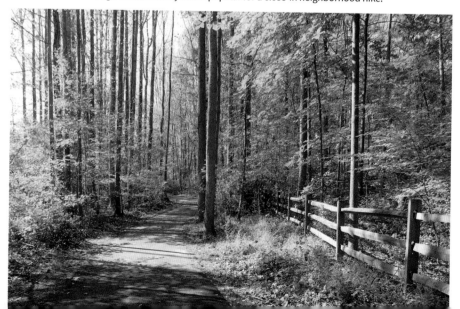

Glade Stream Valley Park

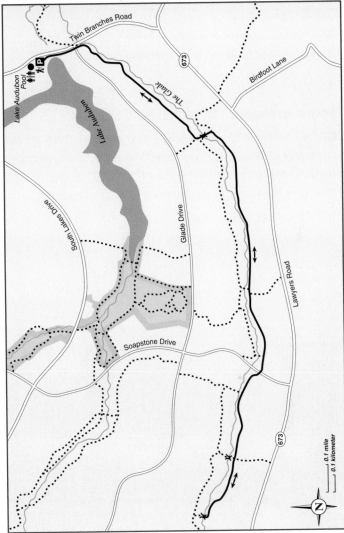

Another option for shortening this hike is to make a loop by turning right on Soapstone Road and then right again on Glade Drive, following Glade Drive back to Twin Branches Road. This route takes you along the road and is not as scenic.

NEARBY/RELATED ACTIVITIES

Visit the Walker Nature Center, (703-476-9689, reston.org) and participate in a variety of educational and recreational programs, such as bird walks, wildlife talks, campfires, and children's programs. The center was named after Reston's first open space and nature center director, Vernon J. Walker, who was hired in 1967. Also, have a picnic or go fishing at Lake Audubon. Drive 3.5 miles to Reston Town Center, and enjoy some shopping or dining at a variety of restaurants.

• •

GPS TRAILHEAD COORDINATES N38° 55.988' W77° 19.548'

> **DIRECTIONS** From the Capital Beltway (I-495), take Exit 45 (VA 267 West) to Exit 14 (Hunter Mill Road). Take Hunter Mill Road left, south, and turn right on Sunrise Valley Drive. Turn left on South Lakes Drive and left again on Twin Branches Road. Lake Audubon Pool is located on the right.

The trail through Glade Stream Valley Park is flat and mostly paved, with a few bridges over the stream.

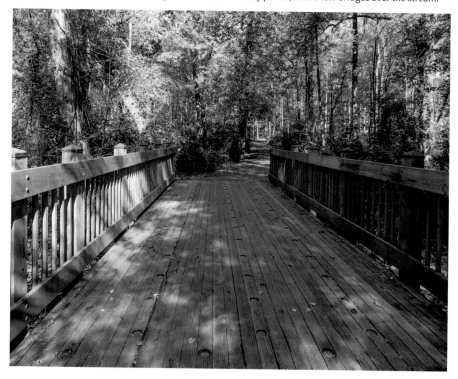

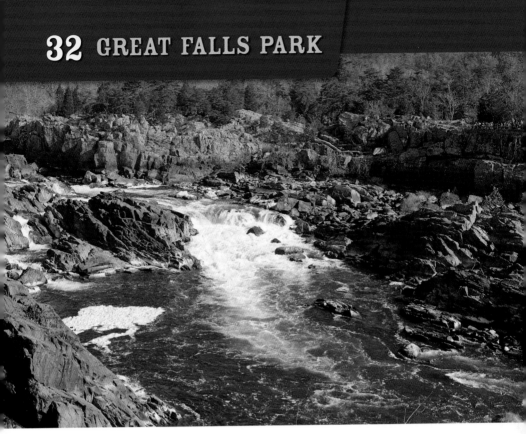

The Great Falls cascade was formed at the fall line on the boundary between the Piedmont Plateau and Atlantic Coastal Plain.

THIS MAGNIFICENT POTOMAC RIVER SETTING in Fairfax County guarantees great falls, great vistas, and a great time. Hikers enjoy a wide array of trails, from extremely challenging to easy and relaxing.

DESCRIPTION

Only 17 miles from the White House, the Great Falls area is probably the metro area's finest close-in natural attraction. The broad and smooth Potomac River suddenly tumbles almost 80 feet in a series of rapids and then squeezes through narrow, mile-long, and sheer-walled Mather Gorge. National Park Service lands protect both banks and provide riveting views of nature at work. On the Virginia side, Great Falls Park stretches the length of the gorge and beyond, and inland to cover 805 acres of rocky shoreline and wooded uplands laced with hiking trails.

This hike is a 5.3-mile figure eight that starts at the falls and travels along the gorge, onto the floodplain, by the historic canal, and close to an aqueduct dam. You're treated to an assortment of scenery, impressive vistas, and about 2,000 feet of elevation change. After parking at the Great Falls Tavern Visitor Center, which is almost always crowded on weekends, begin your hike by following the River Trail,

LENGTH 4.6 miles (with shorter and longer options)

CONFIGURATION Figure-eight loop

DIFFICULTY Easy–difficult

SCENERY Uplands, cliffs, dam, canal, river vistas

EXPOSURE Shady; less so in winter

TRAFFIC Heavy–crowded in falls area on warm-weather weekends and holidays

TRAIL SURFACE Mostly dirt; some pavement and gravel; rocky in places

HIKING TIME 3 hours

DRIVING DISTANCE 20 miles

WHEELCHAIR TRAVERSABLE In some parts

SEASON Year-round

ACCESS Great Falls Park is open daily, sunrise–sunset (closed December 25)

MAPS National Park Service, tinyurl.com/greatfallsmap

FACILITIES Restrooms, water, museum, and phones at visitor center; restrooms and water at Matildaville

CONTACT 703-285-2966, nps.gov/grfa

LOCATION McLean, Virginia

COMMENTS No bikes allowed; dogs must be on leashes; wear good hiking gear and water-proof boots if you plan to hike into the river. The park's fee is $10 per car or $5 per person.

but first make a detour to the first of three overlooks for dynamic views of the magnificent Great Falls. This enormous cascade of water is a 76-foot drop.

The first crowds to visit Great Falls came in 1906, dubbing it the "Niagara of the South." A trolley line was established from Georgetown to the area, passing mostly fields and farms. When trains gave way to automobiles in the 1930s, roads paved the way for suburban growth.

Truly, it's hard to walk away from that first observation deck, but the next overlook is equally stunning, plus you'll see your cohorts across the river in Maryland enjoying their view from Olmsted Island. On any given weekend, Great Falls National Park is nearly "loved to death," as it is overrun with families, dog walkers, serious hikers, photographers, and tourists. Great Falls Park and the C&O Canal across the river are the region's favorite natural landscape. Expect to see picnics, parties, and even weddings; so many people choose to celebrate this natural marvel. However, if you can stop by on a weekday, you'll share the scenery with significantly fewer people.

Continue hiking the River Trail, with its frequent views of the rapids, ravine, and river to your left. On your way to the second overlook, notice the sign indicating flood levels that occurred here in the last century. Returning from the third overlook, turn left and walk about 30 yards to swing onto a twisty clifftop path. Follow it 200 yards, and then swing left to get onto the blue-blazed and rather rocky River Trail. En route, read the information boards and explore some of the unmarked short side trails on the left to peer down into Mather Gorge.

The 200-foot-wide Mather Gorge is a 2-million-year work in progress, being created by the ever-erosive river cutting down through bedrock. At a signage-free intersection, go straight through to cross a stream valley on steep wooden steps.

Great Falls Park

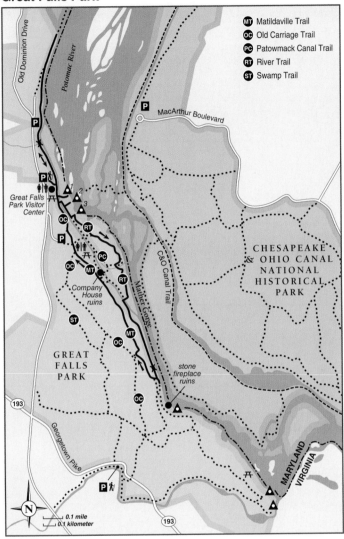

Legend:
- **MT** Matildaville Trail
- **OC** Old Carriage Trail
- **PC** Patowmack Canal Trail
- **RT** River Trail
- **ST** Swamp Trail

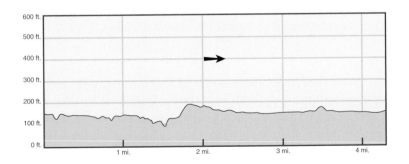

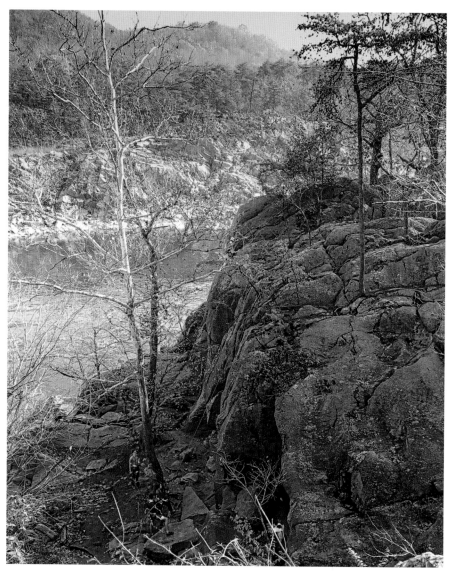

Rock climbing is a popular recreational activity along the cliffs at Great Falls Park.

Continuing, you'll pass several trailside overlooks, and then turn right and inland to cross the old canal bed and reach a T junction. There, turn left and proceed, first passing ruined lock 2 and then passing a deep, man-made rock cleft where locks 3, 4, and 5 once stepped the canal down to the river. Continuing along the gorge, you'll find that the scenery gets wilder, the trail rockier, and the going slower—partly because the moody river requires watching. When unruffled, it glitters harmlessly. But when turbulent, it rushes untamed and intractable.

Frequently there are skilled climbers scaling the gorge, and further below, paddlers. Sometimes it feels like hiking in Great Falls is comparable to Beltway gridlock, so be patient and use extreme caution to avoid twisting an ankle. As you scramble up and over rocks, navigating this uneven terrain, the River Trail makes its way south. Stay away from cordoned-off areas designed to prevent further damage to this fragile ecosystem.

Eventually, the trail opens up and many people quit and head back to the visitor center. Keep going. Continue crossing fields of giant boulders, and then you'll pass a cliff on your right. Footing here is very uneven. When you see the Matildaville Trail signpost, you can make your U-turn, but you might want to walk down to Sandy Landing first to get a fish's-eye view of the river. Sandy Landing is the paved road leading to the river's edge. From down there you realize how huge and high this gorge actually is. Return up the road, and then turn back toward the visitor center following the Old Carriage Trail.

The Old Carriage Trail is wide, flat, and easy to maneuver and soon joins the Matildaville Trail, which takes you through a forest toward the visitor center. You're much higher than the River Trail now, and in the winter, you can see across to the Maryland side. The new-growth forest has lots of colorful beech, oak, and maple trees. You'll pass another intersection, but stay on the Matildaville Trail.

Take a quick detour to see the Company House's rock wall ruins of a house built in the late 1790s by the Patowmack Company. It was intended as housing for the canal superintendent and his family, but the house took so long to build, only one superintendent ever lived there. The canal was one of five waterways built by the Patowmack Company, starting in 1785. The goal was to make the Potomac River navigable and open up waterborne trade with the interior. The company's first president was an ardent advocate named George Washington. After four years, though, he left to become the first president of a larger entity. The Great Falls canal was opened in 1802. For two decades, it had enough boat traffic to support the adjoining town of Matildaville, started by Henry "Light-Horse Harry" Lee. But the company, canal, and town foundered. In 1828 the company's property and rights passed to the Chesapeake & Ohio Canal Company, which tried again on the Maryland side of the river (see Hike 15, page 80). Although ultimately it failed, it left behind what are now some fine hiking venues.

Stay on the gravelly path until you reach the large and exhibit-loaded Great Falls Tavern Visitor Center. Continue on the same path into a grassy open area that was the site of an amusement park a century ago and is now a picnicking area that's thronged with visitors in warm weather. Follow the green blazes and walk north on the Patowmack Canal Trail.

After the visitor center, you'll pass three parking lots on your left and cross over a stream called Mine Run. This is a peaceful trail where you're likely to see abundant wildlife. There are lots of places to walk down to the Potomac, but keep your eye on the aqueduct dam in the distance. The low 19th-century dam that spans the river just below Conn Island feeds Washington's major water-supply intake.

Here, the trail becomes rocky with opportunities to climb out onto the river. For the next mile, you'll experience some of the best riverside hiking ever. Mature sycamores, cottonwoods, and maples, as well as papaws, bushes, and wildflowers, flank the mostly smooth but sometimes muddy trail. Watch for springtime songbirds, summertime butterflies, wintertime water birds, and anytime bald eagles.

When you reach the aqueduct dam, you'll see a sign for Riverbend Park, which is the adjacent national park to the north (see page 174 for hikes). Stop for a short rest on these rocks at the base of the dam before hiking back the way you came toward the Great Falls Tavern Visitor Center.

No bikes are allowed on this trail, but you will see many dogs and kids. It's truly a magical environment that feels far away from civilization and yet is a very short distance from a thriving metropolis.

NEARBY/RELATED ACTIVITIES

Explore other trails, such as Riverbend's Meadow Trail, Difficult Run (Hike 28, page 135), and Great Falls' Matildaville Trail. Linger at Great Falls Tavern Visitor Center to see the nature exhibits. Try one of the many year-round programs the park offers.

• •

GPS TRAILHEAD COORDINATES N38° 59.813' W77° 15.284'

DIRECTIONS From the Capital Beltway (I-495) in McLean, Virginia, take Exit 44 to get onto Georgetown Pike (VA 193) heading roughly west. Stay on the pike 4.2 miles. Then turn right onto Old Dominion Drive. Drive 1 mile and enter Great Falls Park.

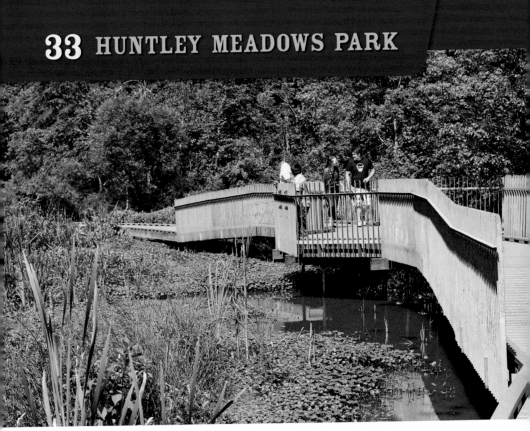

Huntley Meadows is a wonderland for wetland creatures. Stand quietly and you're likely to hear frogs calling to one another or see a snake slither by in the water.

THIS HUGE NATURE PRESERVE in southern Fairfax County is a great place to take a short hike and spend some time observing wildlife, especially birds, frogs, and turtles.

DESCRIPTION

Covering 1,557 acres just south of Alexandria, Huntley Meadows Park celebrated its 40th anniversary in 2016 and ranks as one of the metro area's largest close-in parks. Its centerpiece is a 500-acre freshwater marsh—the area's largest—enveloped by mostly deciduous woodlands. The result is a protected natural habitat with a remarkable array of plants and animals.

The land passed through private and government ownership until President Gerald Ford signed what was then 1,261 acres over to Fairfax County for use as a park in 1975. Under the federal Legacy of Parks program, the county paid only $1 for the land. Ducks Unlimited, a nonprofit supporting wetland preservation, provided financial assistance to Fairfax County Park Authority to purchase an additional 165 acres of adjacent wetland and upland.

LENGTH 2 miles

CONFIGURATION Loop

DIFFICULTY Very easy

SCENERY Wetlands, woodlands

EXPOSURE Mostly shady on the woodland trails. On the boardwalk, there is total exposure. It gets hot in the summer.

TRAFFIC Moderate on weekends, light on weekdays except for birders and school groups on spring mornings

TRAIL SURFACE Mostly fine gravel on main land trails; boardwalk across marsh; dirt on side trails (muddy when wet)

HIKING TIME 2 hours (including time spent looking, listening, and inhaling)

DRIVING DISTANCE 15 miles

SEASON Year-round; best in the warmer months

ACCESS Open daily, sunrise–sunset

WHEELCHAIR TRAVERSABLE On boardwalk, but not on Deer Trail

MAPS USGS *Alexandria, Mount Vernon*

FACILITIES Restroom at parking lot; restrooms, water, and phone at visitor center

CONTACT Visitor center, 703-768-2525; Friends of Huntley Meadows Park, friendsof huntleymeadowspark.org; fairfaxcounty .gov/parks/huntley

LOCATION Alexandria, Virginia

COMMENTS Free brochures available; visitor center is open daily (except Tuesdays), 9 a.m.– 5 p.m. (noon–5 p.m. on holidays). You may want to carry insect repellent during the warm-weather months; Huntley is bug-rich and unsprayed. Also, bring binoculars to see the wildlife. This is such a scenic spot, you will want your smartphone or a camera too.

The helpful signage on the trails explains how this freshwater lowland, carved millions of years ago by the meandering Potomac River, is one of the rarest habitats left in the region. As the signs explain, "Acre for acre, a healthy wetland supports more life than almost any other habitat." They aren't exaggerating—you will see an abundance of wildlife here in every season.

Huntley is an attractive year-round hiking venue, especially for people keen on natural history. But it has only a few maintained trails. Consequently, Huntley hikes tend to be short in distance, although not always in time.

This is a very easy 1.8-mile, hill-less outing using the maintained trails. You'll find that they are in good condition and selectively dotted with useful information boards. Be sure to stay on the trail to avoid both poison ivy and ticks.

To get started from the parking lot, take the 100-yard paved trail to the visitor center. Step inside to check out the exhibits and stock up on flora and fauna checklists and other materials. Also grab a seasonal trail guide from the box outside.

Then get out onto the broad and level Cedar Trail, which heads into the woods for 0.3 mile. With a seasonal trail guide in hand, watch for the numbered trail markers describing interesting facts about the wetlands. At the first trail junction, turn right onto the 0.6-mile Heron Trail, built above the wetlands on a sturdy boardwalk. This vantage point provides ample opportunities to observe nature in action. Just after marker 5, you'll reach the edge of the marsh. From there, staying right, take

Huntley Meadows Park

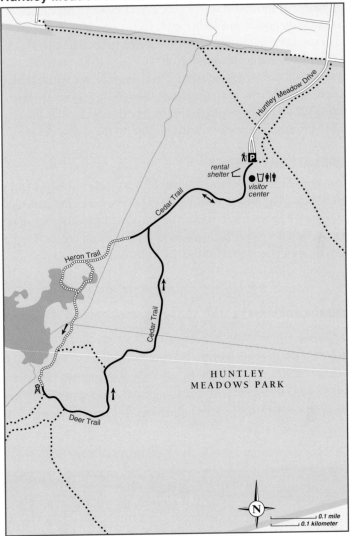

the wooden boardwalk across the wetlands to an observation tower equipped with information boards and great views.

See, hear, read, and even smell what the marsh has to offer. In spring, look and listen for migrating songbirds and mating frogs. In summer, watch for water birds and dragonflies (sometimes they look like moving blossoms on the duckweed-carpeted water), and maybe catch the scent of a common white-plumed plant called lizard's tail. In fall, watch for migrating raptors, warblers, and water birds. In winter, ducks hang around if the marsh doesn't ice over. On warm days, don't be surprised if a black snake slithers past you on the trail, and at any time of year, look for beaver lodges and dams, but don't expect to see the nocturnal builders.

Leaving the observation tower, step off the end of the boardwalk, walk about 15 yards, and turn right onto a dirt side trail. Then, at a junction with a broad woodland trail, turn right to follow the gravel-surfaced Deer Trail. Stay on the main trail at the next junction. Turn right at trail marker 12 to get onto the 1-mile Cedar Trail. Follow Cedar Trail to the next intersection, and continue to the visitor center.

NEARBY/RELATED ACTIVITIES

Explore Huntley's bountiful visitor center, with its nature exhibits and photo-rich display about the park's history. Take advantage of the park's naturalist-led tours and other year-round programs, and try the volunteer-led Monday morning bird walk. Explore the park's hiker/biker trail; get details at the visitor center. The park is about 5 miles from George Washington's Mount Vernon estate.

• •

GPS TRAILHEAD COORDINATES N38° 45.399' W77° 05.917'

> **DIRECTIONS** From the Capital Beltway (I-495) in Alexandria, Virginia, take Exit 177A and follow the long ramp to get onto Richmond Highway (US 1) heading roughly southwest. After 3 miles, turn right onto Lockheed Boulevard. Go 0.7 mile west to the end of Lockheed at Harrison Lane. There, turn left into the park's main entrance and go 0.2 mile to the visitor-center parking lot.

Bird-watchers and naturalist photographers find Huntley Meadows perfect for catching wildlife in action.

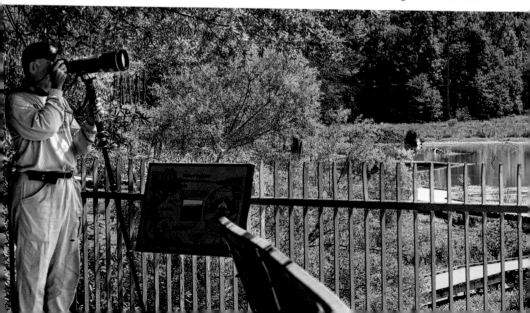

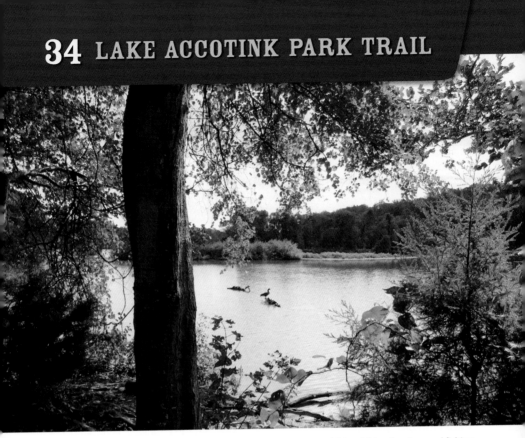

Lake Accotink is a scenic destination for outdoor activities, including hiking, biking, boating, and fishing.

SITUATED ALONG THE CROSS COUNTY TRAIL, Lake Accotink Park has a 4-mile, natural-surface loop trail that runs from the edge of the parking lot below the dam, along the east and north side of the lake, then along Accotink Creek to the Braddock Road underpass. Several information kiosks are located along the trail at connecting trails from residential areas. Other trails stretch beyond the park with extensive options for hiking and mountain biking.

DESCRIPTION

Lake Accotink is a reservoir formed in 1943 by the US Army's damming of Accotink Creek in Fairfax County, Virginia. The lake is surrounded by Lake Accotink Park, which offers a wide range of activities, including bike rentals; canoe and paddleboat rentals; a boat launch; tour boat rides; fishing; a nine-green, double-holed minigolf course; an antique carousel; a snack bar; pavilion shelters and picnic areas with grills; a playground; sand volleyball courts; and basketball courts.

Accotink Trail begins at the main parking lot, which lies atop the longest continuous stretch of surviving roadbed of the Orange and Alexandria Railroad, chartered in 1849 to link the city of Alexandria with Gordonsville in central Virginia. Take the trail on the right side of the parking lot, and cross over the first intersection; then

LENGTH 4.1 miles (with longer options)

CONFIGURATION Loop

DIFFICULTY Easy

SCENERY Lake views, woodlands, neighborhood

EXPOSURE Mostly shady; less so in winter; short open stretch through a neighborhood

TRAFFIC Light; heavier on warm-weather weekends and holidays

TRAIL SURFACE Pavement, dirt, and gravel

HIKING TIME 2 hours

DRIVING DISTANCE 21 miles

SEASON Year-round

ACCESS Open daily, 7 a.m.–sunset

WHEELCHAIR TRAVERSABLE No

MAPS Fairfax County Government, tinyurl.com/lakeaccotinktrailmap

FACILITIES Restrooms at picnic areas and boat-rental area

CONTACT 703-569-3464, fairfaxcounty.gov/parks/lake-accotink

LOCATION Springfield, Virginia

COMMENTS The 493-acre park has many recreational uses and facilities. Swimming, windsurfing, paddleboarding, and gas-powered boat motors are prohibited. A state fishing license is required for fishing. Be aware that the trail section by the dam frequently floods during hard rains and there is no bypass.

head up the steps to see a view of the 55-acre lake. Walk on the trail to the right and follow the steps down toward the beach and boat-rental area. As you pass the carousel on the right, take the trail over the bridge and into the woods on your left. For the rest of the hike, you will continue turning left to walk in a counterclockwise direction, making a complete loop around the lake. The trail signs are pretty easy to follow. Note that the trail is open to bicycles.

When you see a sign for Wakefield Park, turn left to stay on the trail. As you reach the far narrow extensions of the lake, the views become marshland, and you may hear the sounds of wood frogs or American toads and see waterfowl such as blue herons, ducks, and Canada geese. Wildlife thrives on these trails; deer, muskrat, fox, and other critters abound. When you reach mile marker 2, turn left (the trail becomes concrete at this point). The trail connects here to the Gerry Connolly Cross County Trail (Fairfax County's trail system—you could continue north here for a more extensive hike). Cross over the bridge and turn left again, following the signs to return to the marina. To complete the loop, you must walk through a neighborhood for a short distance to reconnect with the Accotink Trail.

The trail ends at Lonsdale Drive as it intersects Danbury Forest Drive. Cross the street and follow the sidewalk past Kings Glen Elementary School. Pass the first entrance to the woods (this goes to a townhouse community), and keep straight across Kirkham Court. Reenter the woods again as you proceed to the trailhead straight ahead, to the right of the playground. At the top of the hill, turn left onto the trail, continuing through the woods 1.4 miles and ending with a steep incline as you return to the dam and the parking lot.

Lake Accotink Park Trail

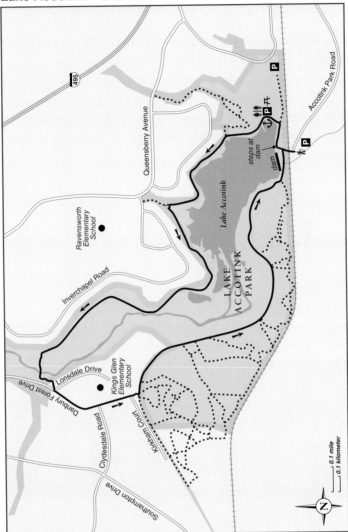

NEARBY/RELATED ACTIVITIES

The Lake Accotink Trail connects to the Gerald Connolly Cross County Trail, which extends 40 miles across the county and offers an extensive venue for hiking or biking. The park is also located just 4.5 miles from Springfield Town Center, a mega shopping destination with a wide range of retailers and dining options.

• •

GPS TRAILHEAD COORDINATES N38° 47.549' W77° 13.076'

DIRECTIONS From the Capital Beltway (I-495), take Exit 54 (Braddock Road/VA 620 East). Go east on Braddock Road, and turn right onto Backlick Road. After passing underneath the interstate, turn right onto Highland Street and then make a slight right onto Accotink Park Road. Turn left to stay on Accotink Park Road. Park in the main parking lot under the railroad bridge.

Visitors can rent paddleboats during the summer months to explore Lake Accotink.

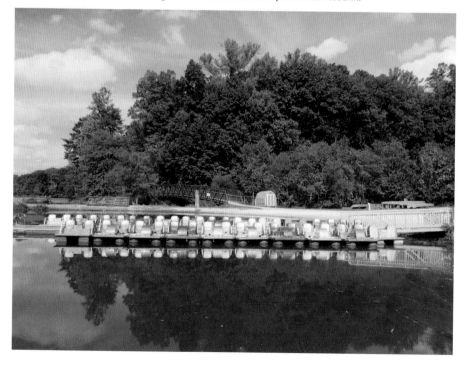

Mason Neck offers a glorious hiking adventure and a favorite habitat for Virginia's bald eagles.

THE STATE PARK and adjoining national wildlife refuge, both on a secluded peninsula in the southeastern corner of Fairfax County, provide a protected habitat for wildlife and some fine woodland and shoreline trails for hikers.

DESCRIPTION

For more than four decades, Mason Neck State Park and Mason Neck National Wildlife Refuge have played a vital role in keeping much of the Mason Neck peninsula green and in helping to restore the area's once-imperiled bald-eagle population. The park and refuge, together with other public lands, now cover most of the 9,000-acre peninsula, which juts into the Potomac River roughly 25 miles southwest of Washington. They are managed cooperatively as a huge nature preserve that also provides humans with recreation opportunities.

Situated between Occoquan and Belmont Bays to the west and the Potomac River to the right, the 1,813-acre park and 2,227-acre refuge consist mostly of rolling woodlands. In 1608 John Smith's exploration party became the first Europeans to see Mason Neck, which had been Moyumpse tribal territory for 350 years. In the late 1600s, the land was occupied by the Mason family, including George Mason IV,

LENGTH 2.4 miles

CONFIGURATION Modified loop

DIFFICULTY Moderate

SCENERY Bay views, marshlands, forest

EXPOSURE Mostly shady; less so in winter

TRAFFIC Usually light; moderate in and near state-park picnic area on warm-weather weekends and holidays

TRAIL SURFACE Mostly dirt, some pavement

WHEELCHAIR TRAVERSABLE Partially

HIKING TIME 2 hours (including beach pauses and marsh gazing)

DRIVING DISTANCE 26 miles

SEASON Year-round, but best from fall through spring

ACCESS State park open daily, 8 a.m.–sunset (entrance fee $5); wildlife refuge open daily, sunrise–sunset

MAPS Virginia Department of Conservation & Recreation, tinyurl.com/masonnecktrailmap

LOCATION Lorton, Virginia

CONTACT Virginia Department of Conservation & Recreation, 703-339-2385, dcr.virginia.gov/state-parks/mason-neck; visitor center, 703-339-2380; refuge office, 703-490-4979; Mason Neck Citizens Association, masonneck.org

FACILITIES Restrooms, water at state-park picnic area; water, phone at state-park visitor center

COMMENTS Swimming, boating, fishing, and camping are allowed. The wildlife-refuge trails are closed December–June.

who built Gunston Hall plantation in the 1750s. This lush landscape was also the site of battles between the British and American colonists during the War of 1812. The location was strategically important, as it served as a shipping channel, but it was ravaged by enemy raids.

The refuge was established in 1969 as the country's first federal sanctuary for bald eagles. The impetus came from the alarming fact that the local eagles (like those elsewhere in the lower 48 states) seemed headed for extinction because of habitat loss and pesticide use. The peninsula was slated for suburban development until the 1960s, when, with significant help from the Nature Conservancy, a public–private coalition helped reverse the situation and preserved what is now the heart of the refuge: the 250-acre Great Marsh. It also contributed to the eagles' comeback (just as nationally the species is no longer listed as endangered). The species' recovery has been remarkable along Virginia's lower Chesapeake Bay and its tidal tributaries, including the Mason Neck area. In 1977 the region had only 33 pairs of eagles (they mate for life); by the spring of 2006, the total had risen to 485 pairs, and by 2010 to more than 680 breeding pairs, concentrated in the lower Chesapeake and Potomac River areas.

The trails are generally well marked and well maintained, with those in the park using color-coded trail names. The trails are only lightly used because nearly all visitors head for the park's waterfront visitor center and nearby picnic area. Be sure to stay on the trails, as some areas are striving to regenerate the woodlands and wildlife. You may want to take along field glasses and a bird book, and remember that winter is the best time to spot waterfowl and eagles.

Mason Neck State Park and National Wildlife Refuge

Although most of the acreage is closed to the public, the modest trail system enables hikers to sample the local scenery, with only about 650 feet of elevation change. Shorter and longer options are available.

To get started, park in the gravel parking lot next to the playground, which is adjacent to the visitor/nature center (pick up a map if needed). The Bay View Trail begins at the kiosk just before the shoreline (other trails, such as Woodthrush and Wilson, have separate parking areas). From the trail you can see a wide swath of the Potomac River. The trail starts out nicely packed and navigable by strollers

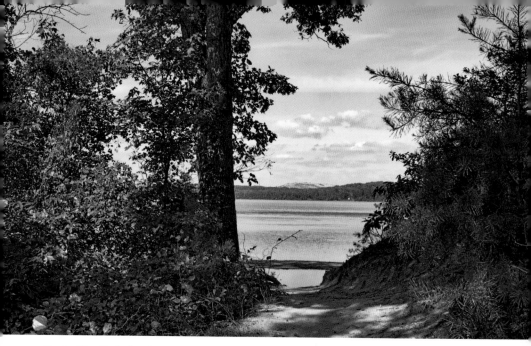

The Bay View Trail offers frequent glimpses of scenic Belmont Bay, which empties into Occoquan Bay and ultimately the Potomac River.

and wheelchairs. As you proceed, you'll come to various overlooks with panoramic views of Belmont Bay. Follow the red blazes through the forest until you come to stairs leading up to the first of several boardwalks built over marshland.

A variety of water-loving plants comes into view, and you'll hear the sound of peeping frogs. Animals and birds can hide among the luxurious tall cattails and water lilies. This marsh is a year-round faunal delight where you'll have a chance to benefit from what Thoreau called "the tonic of wilderness." Ducks, geese, and swans pass through in the spring and fall, with some wintering there. In summer, swallows and other insect eaters cruise the wetland, and herons and egrets dot the marsh like blossoms. The woods shelter migratory songbirds as well as resident birds, deer, and other creatures. They nest and roost in tall trees and roam the local waterways. Starting in November or December, they take six months or more to raise their young.

After you pass the lily pond, you'll enter a thicker part of the forest. At the intersection, take a quick detour to an observation blind, and then return to the intersection. Take the right fork where Bay View joins Wilson Trail. Next you'll pass a bench; then follow the yellow blazes as the trail continues into the forest. You'll pass a second bench and a huge tree that has fallen sideways and is being propped up by another tree. You'll cross over two small bridges on this rooty and shady trail until the forest opens to a parking lot.

The parking lot is adjacent to the main road, which you will cross. Look for the entrance to Kane's Creek Trail, and follow the blue blazes into the forest. At this point, you're likely to hear birds, squirrels, and the rustling of other local wildlife. This is a fragile ecosystem, so don't leave the trail.

At the second intersection, take the center trail (the trail to the right is a 1.3-mile out-and-back option to see Kane's Creek). Follow the blue blazes. You'll continue hiking through the forest until you come to another intersection. Take the trail to the right to stay on the Kane's Creek Trail as it heads back toward the nature center. At the end of this trail you'll pass another kiosk and end up at the parking lot for the nature center. Head to the right of the nature center for one last picturesque view on the Beach Trail. The beginning of the Beach Trail is paved and accommodates strollers, bicycles, or wheelchairs.

There's a little area designated for campfires with benches and beautiful views of the river. Continue to the observation deck, and take a minute to enjoy the scenery. You may see some boats or birds. Then return the way you came and head back to the nature center.

NEARBY/RELATED ACTIVITIES

The visitor center has informative brochures, exhibits, and staff; ask about events and programs, such as the guided canoe trips, both by day and by moonlight. (The center's hours are April–October, weekdays, 10 a.m.–6 p.m.; November–January, weekends, 10 a.m.–5 p.m.; closed in February.) Explore Pohick Bay Regional Park (703-352-5900, novaparks.com), Gunston Hall plantation (703-550-9220, gunston hall.org), and Meadowood Special Recreation Management Area (703-339-3461, tinyurl.com/meadowoodsrma), all of which you'll pass on your drive back along Gunston Road.

• •

GPS TRAILHEAD COORDINATES N38° 38.546' W77° 11.993'

DIRECTIONS From the Capital Beltway (I-495), drive to I-95 South and take Exit 163 to Lorton Road (VA 642). Go left on Lorton Road and head east 1.3 miles. Turn right onto Armistead Road, drive several hundred yards, and then turn right onto Richmond Highway (US 1). Drive 0.8 mile and turn left onto Gunston Road. Proceed generally southeast 4.6 miles. Turn right onto High Point Road and go 1 mile to the contact station (after 0.7 mile, note the refuge trailhead parking lot on the left). Then continue 2 miles to the parking lot at the state-park visitor center. Note: Arrive early on warm-weather weekends and holidays; if the main lot and nearby picnic-area lot are full, walk along the entrance road to the Wilson Spring Trail parking lot, and start hiking from there.

36 POTOMAC OVERLOOK REGIONAL PARK AND NATURE CENTER

After crossing under George Washington Memorial Parkway, you arrive at Potomac Overlook, where you're treated to a panoramic view of the Potomac River.

NESTLED IN THE HEART of Arlington's leafy neighborhoods, this regional park encompasses 67 acres of wild and cultivated land and 2.5 miles of varied trails. Follow interpretive displays to learn about this park and its vegetation. Steep ravines on either side of Donaldson Run lead to the Potomac Heritage Trail (PHT).

DESCRIPTION

This site's human history dates back to 8000 B.C., when hunter-gatherer American Indians roamed the land. Stone bowls found here date back to 2000 B.C., pointing to major Indian occupation. In the mid-1800s, an Italian quarrying community settled at Marcey Creek. Soldiers camped on this land during the Civil War. Eventually, in 1971, the Northern Virginia Regional Park Authority purchased the land from private families to establish and preserve a park for use by the community.

On this easy-to-moderate, hilly suburban hike, you'll crisscross Donaldson Run, a tributary of the Potomac River. The multiple trails are not easy to follow, so definitely print a map or pick one up at the nature center. Most trails branch off from a paved road in the middle of the park, so you can find your way back if you take a wrong turn. To lengthen the hike, take the Donaldson Run Trail to the

LENGTH 2.5 miles (with longer options)

CONFIGURATION Loop plus modified out-and-back

DIFFICULTY Easy–difficult

SCENERY Parklands, stream valleys, ravine

EXPOSURE Mostly shady; less so in winter

TRAFFIC This is a popular urban, neighborhood park used for dog walking, exercising, field trips, summer camp, and family outings.

TRAIL SURFACE Pavement, creek crossings, rocky, dirt

HIKING TIME 1–2 hours

DRIVING DISTANCE 9 miles

SEASON Year-round

ACCESS Park is open daily during daylight hours; nature center is open Tuesday–Saturday, 10 a.m.–5 p.m., and Sunday, 1–5 p.m. (closed on Mondays).

WHEELCHAIR TRAVERSABLE Marcey Road is paved.

MAPS Virginia Regional Park Authority, tinyurl.com/potomacparkmap

FACILITIES Restrooms and parking at Marcey Park entrance; restrooms and maps available at the James Mayer Center for Environmental Education (nature center); organic vegetable garden, birds of prey house, butterfly garden, tennis courts, basketball courts, picnic area, and concert stage

CONTACT NOVA Parks, 703-528-5406, novaparks.com

LOCATION Arlington, Virginia

COMMENTS Overlook Park was named for the trail to the Potomac River that is often closed due to flooding and overgrowth. Do not park at the Donaldson Run private swimming pool lot. You can also access this trail between houses on North 30th Street if you're looking for additional parking.

Potomac River, and walk either south or north on the PHT a few miles. You'll need to return the way you came, as there are no other paths back to the parking lot except Donaldson Run Trail.

The hike route has a few blazes and some useful signs. After parking at the Comfort Station's Marcey Road Park parking lot, walk back down Marcey Road toward the tennis courts. Begin hiking at the trailhead across the street from the Donaldson Run Pool. Although not marked, it's the Tree of Heaven Trail. The trailhead begins in a tangle of thick forest overgrowth, and after 0.1 mile you'll see "Tree of Heaven," an ancient birch tree with an exposed root system.

When you come to the first intersection, at Overlook Trail and White Oak Way, turn left onto Overlook Trail. Unfortunately there are no signs, so use the bench as your landmark. Continue down the ravine. When Overlook Trail dead-ends, turn right onto Donaldson Run Trail, paralleling Donaldson Run.

Through the trees, to your left, you can see North 30th Street and a few houses that back up to the park. After accessing Donaldson Run Trail, you'll have to do a slippery creek crossing, and then cross back over the same creek using a bridge. After you cross the second time, start looking for the yellow blazes. Just use the trail's natural crossing points to follow the trail. Proceed along the Donaldson Run Trail by the creek until you come to the juncture between the Brown Creeper Connector trail that ascends up the hill to the right.

Potomac Overlook Regional Park and Nature Center

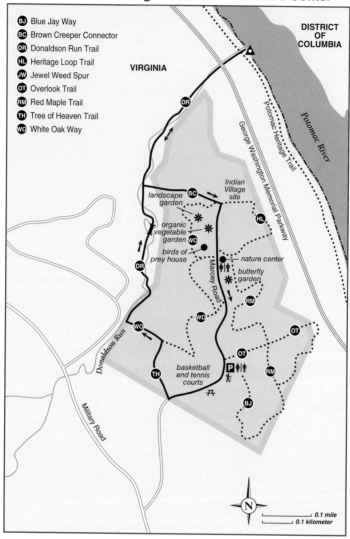

Legend:
- **BJ** Blue Jay Way
- **BC** Brown Creeper Connector
- **DR** Donaldson Run Trail
- **HL** Heritage Loop Trail
- **JW** Jewel Weed Spur
- **OT** Overlook Trail
- **RM** Red Maple Trail
- **TH** Tree of Heaven Trail
- **WO** White Oak Way

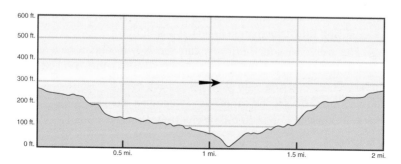

To lengthen the hike, continue straight ahead on the Donaldson Run Trail until you pass under George Washington Memorial Parkway. After about 0.2 mile you'll reach the Potomac Heritage Trail that travels the length of the Potomac River on the Virginia side. Here you can turn right to walk south or left to walk north on the Potomac Heritage Trail for serene views of the Potomac River. At the end of Donaldson Run Trail, turn around and head back. You'll need to scramble over several obstacles to return to the intersection. At the intersection, marked with signs, turn left and follow the Brown Creeper Connector up the hill.

The mulched Brown Creeper Connector has steps that ascend to the Jewelweed Spur. Go right at Jewelweed Spur and you'll pass a playground and sculpture that looks like a spider. Shortly the trail turns into a paved road used by ranger vehicles and becomes Marcey Road. Continue up the paved road, and on your right is the enclosed organic vegetable garden, which is fenced in to keep the deer out. There's also an adjacent garden with native shade plants and a small pond filled with bullfrogs in the summer.

Along that same road, you'll pass the birds of prey house and then the nature center. If it's open, stop at the nature center to explore the Energerium, a collection of interactive exhibits on nature and energy. There is also a library and multiple live-animal enclosures housing snakes, toads, and turtles.

NEARBY/RELATED ACTIVITIES

The park has tennis and basketball courts, a butterfly garden, and a nature center. Nearby, visit Arlington National Cemetery (arlingtoncemetery.mil) to pay your respects to the fallen soldiers and dignitaries laid to rest there. Stop at historic Arlington House (nps.gov/arho) for a tour of the property that once belonged to Robert E. Lee's wife, Mary Custis Lee.

• •

GPS TRAILHEAD COORDINATES N38° 54.704' W77° 06.463'

DIRECTIONS From the U.S. Capitol, take I-395 South from Independence Avenue to George Washington Memorial Parkway. Drive 5.2 miles and take the Spout Run Parkway exit. Continue west on North Spout Run Parkway to Lorcom Lane, and take a right. Take another right on Nelly Custis Drive, and turn right again on Marcey Road, 2.1 miles from Spout Run Parkway.

From the East Falls Church or Ballston Metro, take either Metrobus 15L or ART Bus 53. There are bike lanes on Military and Marcey Roads. For more information, contact Metro, 202-637-7000, wmata.com.

The Potomac Heritage Trail is an ideal environment for those who love scenic riverside hiking.

ENJOY WOODLAND, POND, AND RIVER VISTAS and a family-friendly experience in this grand Potomac River setting in Fairfax County.

DESCRIPTION

Only about 20 miles from the White House, Riverbend Park and its neighbor, Great Falls Park, are probably some of the metro area's finest close-in natural attractions. Fairfax County's 409-acre Riverbend Park is a popular place to kayak, with wooded uplands, hiking trails, and a pretty floodplain shoreline.

This hike is a double-loop walk that accesses part of the Potomac Heritage Trail (PHT), along the Potomac River, as well as a few moderate climbs through dense forests. You'll experience openings in the path with views of the fast-moving Potomac River, but keep your distance; do not try to wade or swim here. The route has limited blazes and signposts, so follow the directions closely—and avoid the poison ivy.

The Riverbend Visitor Center, an interactive museum, explains the geology of the area, specifically the evolution of the tectonic plates and their role in creating the geography here. It also contains a hollowed-out boat used by the American Indian

LENGTH 3.2 miles (with shorter options)

CONFIGURATION Double loop

DIFFICULTY Moderate

SCENERY Uplands, river vistas

EXPOSURE Shady; less so in winter

TRAFFIC Usually light, but can be crowded on warm-weather weekends and holidays

TRAIL SURFACE Mostly dirt; some pavement and gravel; rocky in places

HIKING TIME 3 hours

DRIVING DISTANCE 23 miles

SEASON Year-round

ACCESS Riverbend Park entrance is free and open daily at 7 a.m.; closes seasonally 5–8:30 p.m.

MAPS Available in the visitor center; tinyurl .com/rbtrailmap

WHEELCHAIR TRAVERSABLE No

FACILITIES Restrooms, water, visitor center, concessions, boating rentals, nature center, two parking lots.

CONTACT Riverbend Park, 703-759-9018, www.co.fairfax.va.us/parks/riverbend; Great Falls Park, 703-285-2966 or nps.gov/grfa

LOCATION Great Falls, Virginia

tribes who inhabited this region. There is a gift shop, and usually a ranger is on duty to help direct you to different attractions and to provide maps.

From Riverbend Park, it's also popular to walk south to Great Falls, but for this hike we have chosen to proceed north because it is less traveled. There is ample parking by the Riverbend Visitor Center. To get started, walk down to the riverbank and look left. You'll see an undulating dirt path, part of the PHT, through the trees heading north. The trail, designated with green blazes, will take you through the heavily wooded stream valleys; occasional benches offer rest as you watch wildlife.

For the next 0.4 mile you'll experience some of the best riverside hiking in the area. You'll be on the floodplain where the Potomac makes the big bend for which the park is named. You'll be on the PHT and simultaneously on the Potomac Gorge Interpretive Trail. American elm, hackberry, butternut, sycamore, hickory, cotton-wood, maple, and papaw trees (some identified with small signs) flank the mostly smooth but sometimes muddy trail. Shrubs and wildflowers also line the trail. Keep an eye out for wildlife, including foxes, turtles, bullfrogs, and gophers. Watch for springtime songbirds, summertime butterflies, wintertime water birds, and bald eagles (they live on Conn Island—and unusually far inland for eagles).

Keep going on the heavily papaw-lined trail, and you'll come to a sign pointing out the nature center. Here's where you leave the PHT and turn left toward the nature center. If you prefer, rather than leave this trail you may continue up the PHT for as many more miles as you can handle, then double back. For this hike, we chose to walk uphill on a rocky path following the Hollows Trail's orange blazes. The dirt path ascends steeply 0.2 mile and eventually becomes a gravel path. Turn right when the trail splits, and take the wooden stairs on the connector trail to the nature center.

Riverbend Park and the Potomac Heritage Trail Network

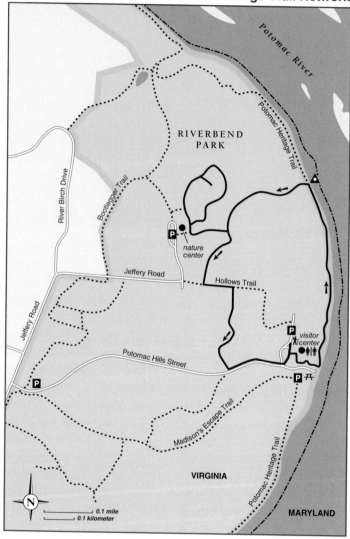

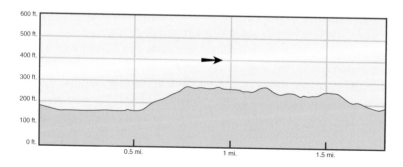

The nature center is open for events, but it has a paved trail called the Duff N Stuff Loop that families with children in strollers or people with disabilities can use to walk through the forest. There are also habitats and cages for injured animals. There's a wooden bridge to cross, and the ground cover in the summer is thick with lush ferns and sassafras bushes.

After returning to the nature center, look for the sign pointing to the Riverbend Visitor Center; follow the orange blazes. The route stays on higher ground through the trees. When you arrive at a semipaved, semidirt road, head left or down toward the river. Make a quick right on Hollows Trail. You can either take Hollows Trail on another loop or return to the visitor center by taking Potomac Hills Road toward the river.

An optional shorter hike begins at the nature center parking lot. Look for the opening of the Lake Trailhead at the edge of the parking lot. The Lake Trail starts out in the woods and descends to lower ground on the Bootlegger Trail. You will cross a bridge over a small stream and continue on a wooden path. Follow the red blazes over rolling terrain until you see a verdant pool named Carpers Pond. You may hear the bullfrogs calling to one another here while dragonflies skim the surface. A sign describes the wildlife, including raccoons, frogs, beetles, turtles, wood ducks, and moles, all of which depend on this habitat. After reading the sign, you can either return up the hill or proceed toward the sound of the rushing Potomac. If you continue your descent, you'll come to an intersection of the Lake Trail and the PHT. Just below this is an opening to see the river and huge boulders on the right flanking the riverbank. From the PHT you can see Gladys Island. Return the way you came.

NEARBY/RELATED ACTIVITIES

Great Falls Park (703-757-3101, nps.gov/grfa; $10 fee per car), on the Virginia side of the Potomac, has several hiking trails, including the PHT, which parallels the river and leads to Riverbend Park. You're only a few miles from Tysons Corner Center I and II. Clemyjontri Park (703-388-2807, fairfaxcounty.gov/parks/clemyjontri) is a fabulous interactive playground for small children, including those with disabilities.

• •

GPS TRAILHEAD COORDINATES N39° 01.116' W77° 14.768'

DIRECTIONS From the Capital Beltway (I-495) in McLean, Virginia, take Exit 44 to get onto Georgetown Pike (VA 193) heading roughly west. Stay on the pike 4.7 miles. Then turn right onto River Bend Road (VA 603). Drive 2.2 miles and turn right onto Jeffery Road (VA 1268). Proceed 1.3 miles, past Riverbend Park's main entrance, to the parking lot at the end of the gated road, next to the park's former nature center.

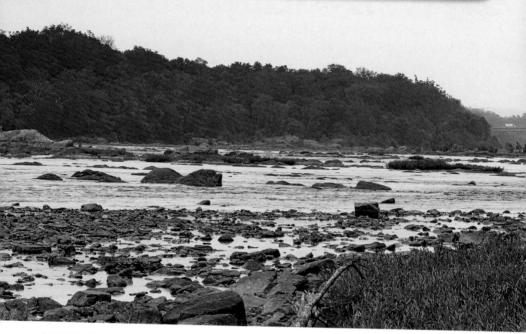

Scott's Run is a popular hike for families, runners, and dog walkers. From the Potomac River, you can see the American Legion Bridge that crosses from Fairfax County into Montgomery County.

OUT-OF-SIGHT SCOTT'S RUN NATURE PRESERVE, on the Potomac River very near the beltway, is well supplied with flora, fauna, breathtaking cliff and river views, a waterfall, and rapids, with a variety of hiking trails.

DESCRIPTION

Hidden amid upscale subdivisions in Fairfax County, Scott's Run Nature Preserve consists of a hilly tract of riverside woodlands scarcely 4 crow-miles northwest of Washington. For songbirds and other wildlife, it's a sanctuary. For locals, it's a community park. And for hikers, it's one of the metro area's loveliest close-in venues. For years, owner Edward Burling used the area as a weekend getaway while allowing hikers to roam his almost 400 acres. After he died, the tract was sold to a developer. But in 1970, local residents and officials managed to fold it into the county's park system.

This hike loops through thickly wooded uplands and reaches the river in three places. It's hilly enough to provide about 420 feet of elevation change. There are trailside maps, and blazes are usually easy to spot, but take a map and plan your route before you go. Also, watch for signs on the Potomac Heritage Trail, which traverses the shoreline; it can be muddy, rooty, and rocky. Note that riverside trails can be tricky or even hazardous when wet or icy. The cliffs over the rapids, more so.

LENGTH 3 miles (with shorter or longer options)

CONFIGURATION Two loop trails

DIFFICULTY Easy–difficult

SCENERY Rolling woodlands, shoreline, waterfall, river views

EXPOSURE Mostly shady; less so in winter

TRAFFIC Moderate on main path to river, especially on warm-weather evenings, weekends, and holidays; elsewhere, usually light

TRAIL SURFACE Mostly dirt or gravel; rocky and rooty near river, with some cliffs

HIKING TIME 2.5 hours (including dawdle-at-river time)

DRIVING DISTANCE 15 miles

SEASON Year-round

ACCESS Open daily, sunrise–sunset

WHEELCHAIR TRAVERSABLE In parts, if wheelchair has mountain bike–style tires

MAPS Posted at trailhead and at many trail intersections; tinyurl.com/scottsruntrailmap

FACILITIES None

CONTACT Nearby Riverbend Park, 703-759-9018

LOCATION McLean, Virginia

COMMENTS Scott's Run is polluted, so don't touch the water.

To get started, park at the Scott's Run eastern parking lot. Take the purple trail, also known as the Parking Lot Connector Trail, to the left. Proceed along a winding and undulating dirt trail that roughly parallels Georgetown Pike. After passing two side trails on the right, bear left at a fork and cross an eroded gully. You'll come to a set of wooden steps to the Scott's Run western parking lot. Go down the wooden steps to the gravel parking lot, and look for the trailhead for the blue path along the creekbed that leads to Scott's Run Waterfall. While at the parking lot, check out the billboard that describes the geography of Scott's Run Nature Preserve.

Head down the narrow, curving trail marked with blue blazes. It is considered part of the Potomac Heritage Trail on the Scott's Run map, though the trail doesn't parallel the river. Instead, it follows Scott's Run, a rushing, bubbling creek, to the Potomac. This nature preserve is part of a rare ecosystem known as the Potomac Gorge, and it offers hikers the chance to experience a unique landscape in Fairfax County.

For the most part, the blue trail is flat and a straight shot toward the falls, except for two creek crossings. When the water level is medium to high, use caution as you cross, walking on the concrete stepping posts built for this purpose.

Next you'll pass a trail that heads over a bridge and into the woods. This trail leads to the Burling Cabin site on Burling Cabin Trail (green blazes). If you're curious, it's just a short walk to the cabin. Otherwise, keep following the blue blazes to the shoreline. The next intersection has steps that turn slightly right and a sign pointing to Scott's Run Waterfall to the left. The sign at the steps describes how local residents saved 336 acres of the preserve from being developed into a subdivision.

Make your way down the rocky path toward a clearing and a wide opening to the Potomac River. Here, beneath a great arc of open sky, you'll find a stretch of

Scott's Run Nature Preserve

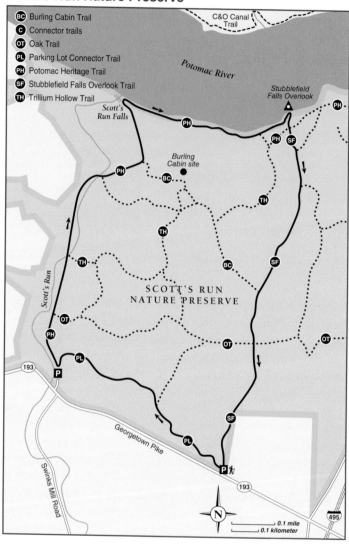

BC Burling Cabin Trail
C Connector trails
OT Oak Trail
PL Parking Lot Connector Trail
PH Potomac Heritage Trail
SF Stubblefield Falls Overlook Trail
TH Trillium Hollow Trail

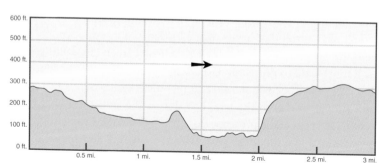

unspoiled Potomac shoreline. Over on the Maryland shore, in the Carderock area, lurks part of the Billy Goat Trail. In the river are the shoals known as Stubblefield Falls. Along with views of a magnificent waterfall, start looking for wildlife here, especially birds such as eagles, egrets, and hawks. Walk out on the peninsula to enjoy a view of the Cabin John Bridge to the right and numerous islands to the left. Enjoy additional fine river views and reach a lovely waterfall-fed, rock-enclosed pool at the mouth of Scott's Run. But resist the temptation to swim or wade; it's against the law because storm runoff pollutes the water.

After enjoying the view, retrace your steps until you see the rooty, uneven blue trail that turns left along the shoreline of the Potomac River. From here, follow the signs designating the rocky, narrow Potomac Heritage Trail, with frequent river views to the left and imposing cliffs along the right side. Continue heading upriver on this narrow trail that is somewhat overgrown. The trail soon becomes a rocky and rooty path that angles uphill, crosses a rock-slab streambed, and skirts the base of a huge rock.

About 60 yards beyond the rock, stop at the first of several spots that offer gorgeous views. It's a one-person, fern-fringed overlook just a few steps off the trail. Next you'll come to the intersection of several trails, including a connector that leads to Stubblefield Falls Overlook. Climb up the cliffs to get a stunning view of the rapids below and multiple islands on the Potomac River. The cliffs are very steep, but don't be surprised to see kids and dogs climbing around.

When you're ready to head back, go south, following the yellow-blazed Stubblefield Falls Overlook Trail. This gradual ascent is slow and long, but once you've made it to the top, just keep following the yellow blazes back to the eastern parking lot.

NEARBY/RELATED ACTIVITIES

Farther west along Georgetown Pike, explore Great Falls Park (703-757-3101, nps.gov/grfa) and Riverbend Park (703-759-9018, www.co.fairfax.va.us/parks /riverbend. To see the same area from a different vantage point, take I-495 to the Maryland side, and follow the signs for Carderock Recreation Area. You can access the Billy Goat Trail from the C&O Canal towpath. If you're hungry, you're just a few miles from Tysons Corner mall area, with its dozens of restaurants and shops.

• •

GPS TRAILHEAD COORDINATES N38° 57.395' W77° 11.902'

DIRECTIONS From the Capital Beltway (I-495) in McLean, Virginia, take Exit 44 to get onto Georgetown Pike (VA 193) heading roughly west. Proceed 0.5 mile and look for the sign on the right. Turn into the preserve's eastern parking lot. If the lot is full, continue up the pike to the western lot, and start the hike there.

39 TURKEY RUN PARK AND THE POTOMAC HERITAGE TRAIL

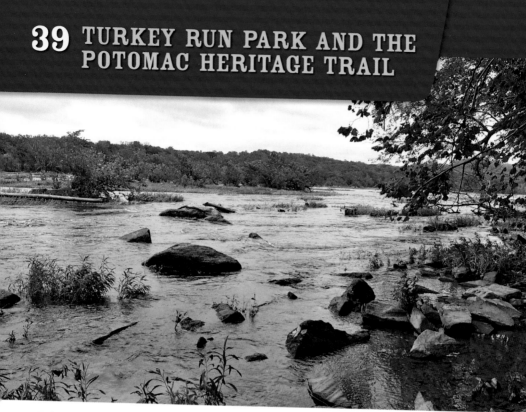

Turkey Run is a segment of the National Park Service's Potomac Heritage Trail. Though just a few miles from urban sprawl, the hike feels like deep wilderness.

FAIRFAX COUNTY IS THE CLOSE-IN HOME of a far-out trail through woodland forest, with fairly steep climbs down and back up from the Potomac River. The trail offers scenic river views, wilderness, and recreational facilities.

DESCRIPTION

Turkey Run Park consists of 700 pristine acres of mature, second-growth upland forest. This rich environment once nurtured Indian tribes living on the banks of the Potomac River. During the Civil War, Union troops occupied the area to protect the Federal City. This verdant deciduous forest is an ideal habitat for reptiles, bats, beavers, foxes, and white-tailed deer. Called the Potomac Gorge ecosystem, the terraced park offers a memorable hiking experience from the uplands down to the water's edge. The park offers picnic areas, limited recreational facilities, and ample parking, but once you've stepped onto the vertical trails, you'll feel worlds away from the city.

Start your hike on the Turkey Run Loop trailhead, located at the edge of parking lot C. There's a sign with a map of the recreation area there. Begin by hiking down wooden stairs to the Potomac River. Keep a lookout for the yellow blazes, as there are two options. You can take the easier trail to the left, but we descended on the loop trail, which is a bit steeper.

LENGTH 2.6 miles

CONFIGURATION Loop

DIFFICULTY Moderate–difficult

SCENERY River views, woodlands, waterfalls, forest

EXPOSURE Shady; less so in winter

TRAFFIC Usually light; busier on weekends and holidays

TRAIL SURFACE Mostly dirt, with rooty, grassy, rocky, and muddy stretches; a few boulder climbs; hills

HIKING TIME 1.5–2 hours

DRIVING DISTANCE 12 miles

SEASON Year-round

ACCESS Open 6 a.m.–10 p.m., but the picnic area closes at 4:15 p.m. on weekdays and all weekend.

WHEELCHAIR TRAVERSABLE No

MAPS National Park Service, tinyurl.com/turkeyrunmap

FACILITIES Restrooms, water, and picnic tables; water and restrooms are not available October–April.

CONTACT National Park Service, 703-289-2500, nps.gov/gwmp; Potomac Heritage National Scenic Trail office, nps.gov/pohe; Potomac Heritage Trail Association, potomactrail.org

LOCATION McLean, Virginia

Through the woods, you will catch glimpses of the Potomac River and realize you're quite high above it, around 350 feet from the shoreline. Despite the feeling of isolation in this wild natural environment, there's still plenty of road noise from the various highways that pass near this park.

As you get closer to the river, you'll see fast-moving rapids, along with islands and fertile marshland. The scene is truly magnificent. Hold the guardrails because the steps are uneven with protruding roots. Next you'll come to a bench with a panoramic—if somewhat obscured by trees—view of the shoreline.

Near the bottom of the hill, the sign for the Potomac Heritage Trail (PHT) is posted. It lists distances to the American Legion Bridge to the left, and Theodore Roosevelt Island and Chain Bridge to the right. Turn right, south, here, and begin following the PHT as it skirts the rocky coast of the Potomac River. Stop at the regular overlooks for dramatic views of the river. You may see a heron, seagull, duck, or raptor, as this is prime habitat for waterfowl, birds of prey, and shorebirds.

In late spring, summer, or early fall, wildflowers grow along the trail. It is very narrow, with rocks and boulders, ferns, and fallen trees housing entire colonies of forests. As you pass a ravine to your right, it appears that a rockslide occurred, knocking down other huge trees. Stay on the PHT by following the occasional blue blaze.

When you come to a huge mound of falling rocks on the shoreline, there's a large rock to climb for a panoramic view of the river from every direction. Notice the tiny island to the right; this is a wonderful place to sit and relax and have a snack. After this, the trail becomes quiet and you can only hear sounds of the river. Look across the river to see Glen Echo Park and MacArthur Boulevard in the District.

Turkey Run Park and the Potomac Heritage Trail

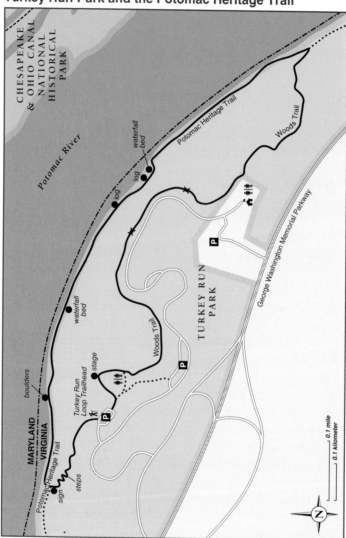

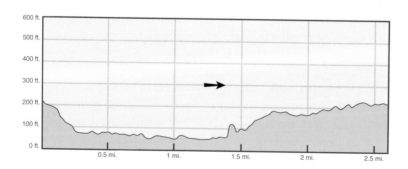

You'll pass two waterfall beds, which may or may not contain water depending on recent rainfall. After the second waterfall, the trail transitions away from the shoreline and heads deeper into the woods. The third waterfall bed has rushing water. Directly after, you'll come to a concrete floodplain-measurement pole with a blue blaze on it. Just around the bend, turn right on the Woods Trail to climb back up the hill. As you climb, you'll see the George Washington Memorial Parkway headquarters with restrooms and picnic tables. Stay on the Woods Trail marked with red blazes. It meanders around area B and then eventually leads you back to parking lot C. There's a second restroom at parking lot C.

NEARBY/RELATED ACTIVITIES

Don't miss the Claude Moore Colonial Farm (703-442-7557, 2017.1771.org). It's a fully immersive living history museum with actors portraying life on a farm circa 1771. For a small fee, you can wander around the farm, see ducks and chickens, and interact with the actors speaking the dialect of the time. For additional hiking, just south of Turkey Run on the George Washington Memorial Parkway is Theodore Roosevelt Island (page 52). North of Turkey Run is Scott's Run (page 178).

• •

GPS TRAILHEAD COORDINATES N38° 57.853' W77° 09.188'

DIRECTIONS Take I-495 to Exit 43 and merge onto the George Washington Memorial Parkway. Head south until you come to the exit for Turkey Run Park. Go left at the sign on the exit ramp to enter the park. If you're heading north on the GW Parkway, take the exit for Turkey Run Park, and turn right at the sign to enter the park.

Walk down these steps to reach the banks of the Potomac River.

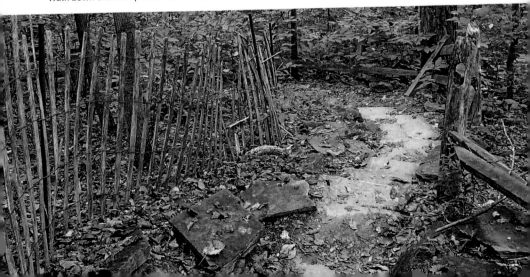

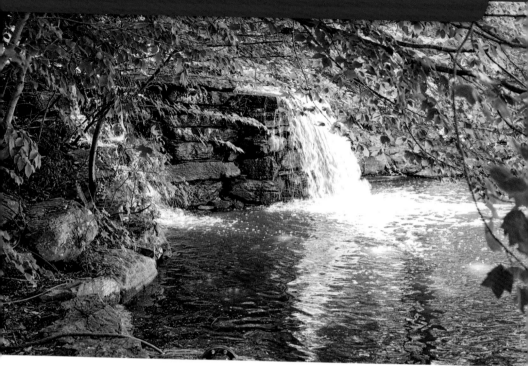

This small urban park is perfect for families with young children seeking a quick jaunt through the woods.

A PRIVATE NATURE SANCTUARY hidden in western Alexandria, Winkler Botanical Preserve is a lovely and unusual place to take a mini hike in the city while feeling like you are far from it.

DESCRIPTION

The Winkler Botanical Preserve is an extraordinary urban locale. Despite being surrounded by apartment complexes and office buildings, the enclosed park is a tranquil place that seems to be part wilderness and part campground. The scenery varies every few yards, and within the 44 acres lie gentle wooded hills, a full-size mountain lodge, a small lake, a half-hidden pond, several little streams, a miniature waterfall, mini meadows, a wooden bridge, and a small-scale network of trails.

In the mid-1970s, the property was an overgrown and refuse-strewn tract of neglected land along Shirley Memorial Highway. Its transformation began later that decade, when the Mark Winkler family decided to create a private botanical preserve.

It had to be built literally from below ground. The terrain itself was reshaped. Vast amounts of stone were trucked in to give the rock-poor tract some outcrops and character. An integrated lake, pond, and stream system was created to control erosion and enhance the landscape. The Winkler family decided that, as both a

LENGTH 0.9 mile

CONFIGURATION Loop

DIFFICULTY Very easy

SCENERY Small-scale woodlands, meadows, lake, pond, streams

EXPOSURE Shady; less so in winter

TRAFFIC Very light–light; increases to moderate when school groups visit

TRAIL SURFACE Mostly wood-chip mulch or mulch and dirt; some gravel, grass

HIKING TIME 1–2 hours (including dawdling)

DRIVING DISTANCE 10 miles

SEASON Year-round but best in warm-weather and leafy months; groups of up to

5 people can visit whenever the preserve is open; larger groups are limited to weekdays and must call to make reservations.

ACCESS Open daily, 8:30 a.m.–5 p.m. (but closed on major holidays)

WHEELCHAIR TRAVERSABLE No

MAP USGS *Alexandria*

FACILITIES None

CONTACT 703-578-7888

LOCATION Alexandria, Virginia

COMMENTS Remember that entrance gates close at 5 p.m.; stay on trails to avoid trampling vegetation; observe posted regulations.

sanctuary and a research and educational institution, the preserve would specialize in plants native to the Potomac River valley. So old trees were saved, alien plants were removed, and a long-term effort was begun to plant hundreds of native species. Catherine Lodge (named for a Winkler) was built to serve as the preserve's headquarters and as a meeting place for nature-oriented classes and other programs aimed at both schoolchildren and families.

Today, the preserve has a few recreational structures, including a ropes course and climbing wall. It is a reflection of what nature and conservation-minded people can achieve in concert, despite the crush of urbanization built literally up to the fences.

It also has 70 species of trees and about 650 species of wildflowers and other plants. Its resident and transient wildlife population includes red foxes, small mammals and rodents, red-shouldered hawks, and lots of other birds. This 0.9-mile hike uses some of the preserve's trails, which, although well maintained, are neither signposted nor blazed. Nor are the plants labeled. So if you're botanically curious, take along some reference books. Do the same if you're interested in birds, as they're not labeled either.

The preserve is at its best during the warm-weather months, when tree leaves hide the nearby buildings, and the frog and insect chorus masks some of the traffic noise. It's a wonderful place for introducing young kids to both nature and hiking. But make sure that everyone stays on the trail—and that the family dog stays home.

To get started, from the parking lot, step onto the preserve's gravel-surfaced main path, and follow it about 200 yards to the lodge. The lodge is open only when the camp is in session or there is a designated event, so don't try to go in or expect

Winkler Botanical Preserve

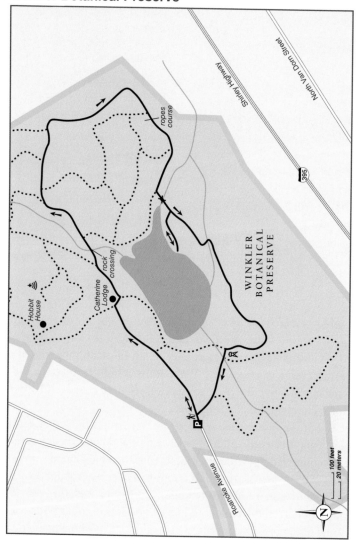

to find a bathroom, but do try out the unusually comfortable wooden bench next to the path.

As you proceed toward the lodge, you'll see a sign describing the rules for using this park. In the summer, the mulched path is bordered by wildflowers, including Queen Anne's lace, daisies, buttercups, and bluebells.

There are two paths. One passes through a wooden gateway and proceeds uphill on a dirt trail. After passing a small rock pool, you'll reach a simple wooden structure that the preserve's staff calls the Hobbit House. Another option is to head right, toward the 2-acre pond that is landscaped with water lilies, lotus flowers, cattails, and other plants. You'll see a man-made waterfall in the distance. We chose the path to the right, which you will see on the map provided. Unfortunately, there is no trail map or any blazes to follow, so this is a free-flowing meander through the woods. The entire park is small enough that you can detour and circle back without losing much ground. All the paths cross over one another at various points, and the entire preserve is quite compact, so feel free to choose whatever path intrigues you.

As you walk down the path, there is a stream to your left, and you'll see clearings where campers meet—a woodland classroom consisting of a small amphitheater. Follow the trail uphill to a wooden bench. This is the steepest part of the trail and the path is rocky and uneven here, so be careful. All around you are lush forests of native trees such as tulip, oak, and hickory. As the path turns downhill, you'll come to a wooden bridge and a waterfall. Cross the bridge, and follow the path that borders the lake. Continue on the path, and take a detour to investigate the waterfall up close. From here, return to the trail and head uphill, where you'll see mountain laurel and rhododendrons beside the rocky path. The trail splits again, and you can continue back to the entrance or take another detour to the climbing tower and observation deck. To return to your car, head left toward the trailhead—and be sure to do so by 4:30 p.m.

NEARBY/RELATED ACTIVITIES

You can combine this hike with Huntley Meadows (Hike 33, page 157). It's also close to Fort Ward Museum & Historic Site (703-746-4848, alexandriava.gov/fortward), a Civil War military museum with a well-preserved battlefield, cannons on display, a playground, an amphitheater, and a picnic area. You're also a few miles from Old Town Alexandria, which is worth a visit for its charming shops and restaurants.

• •

GPS TRAILHEAD COORDINATES N38° 49.659' W77° 07.403'

DIRECTIONS From Washington, cross the Potomac River and head southwest on Shirley Memorial Highway (I-395) about 5.4 miles. Get off at Exit 4 and turn right onto Seminary Road. Drive northwest 0.2 mile. At the second traffic light, turn left onto North Beauregard Street. Proceed 0.9 mile, counting off side streets on the left; take the fifth one, Roanoke Avenue. Follow it 0.1 mile and drive through the gated entrance into the preserve's parking lot at 5400 Roanoke Ave. If the lot is full, park along the avenue outside the gates.

Or use the local bus service and your feet to get to the preserve— Metrobus and DASH operate along North Beauregard Street, and Roanoke Avenue has sidewalks. Contact Metro, 202-637-7000, wmata.com; or DASH, 703-370-3274 or dashbus.com.

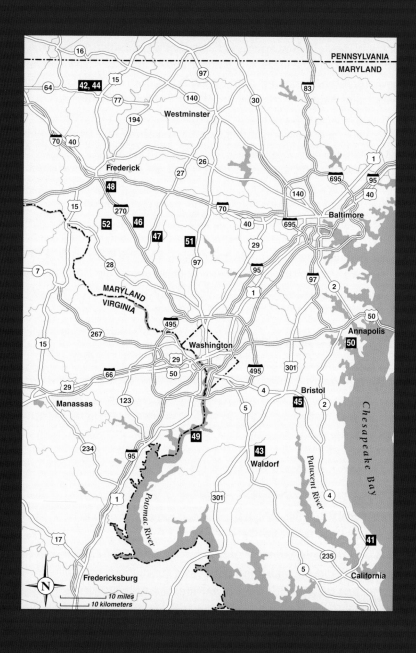

RURAL MARYLAND
(Parts of Montgomery and Prince George's Counties; Anne Arundel, Calvert, and Frederick Counties)

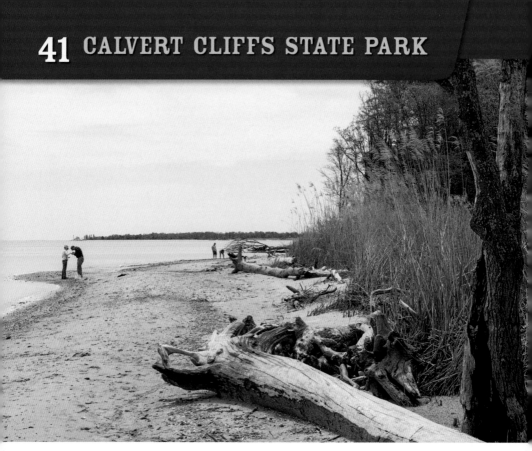

The beachfront park is a popular destination for fossil hunting.

FAMOUS FOR THE ABUNDANCE OF FOSSILS and prehistoric shark teeth found along the sandy beaches of the Chesapeake Bay, Calvert Cliffs State Park is a popular destination for hikers and beachcombers alike. The main hiking trail to the beach offers visitors a wonderland of almost mystical beauty as it passes through wetlands and forest.

DESCRIPTION

Surprisingly, finding an ancient shark's tooth is a common occurrence on this stretch of land—the western shoreline of Maryland's Chesapeake Bay. Although the friendly park rangers at Calvert Cliffs State Park will help you find one, most of the fun is in the search. This 1,400-acre park in southern Maryland features beaches flanked by sedimentary cliffs dating back to the Miocene era, about 6–20 million years ago. As these cliffs erode, more than 600 species of prehistoric treasures keep miraculously tumbling onto the water's edge waiting to be discovered.

People can access the beach either by boat or by hiking the trails leading to the shoreline. The most direct route is the Red Trail, a 1.8-mile trek from the Calvert Cliffs State Park entrance. Along the way, you'll pass protected marshlands peppered

LENGTH 3.7 miles

CONFIGURATION Modified loop (with shorter and longer options)

DIFFICULTY Easy–moderate

SCENERY Woodlands, wetlands, marsh, beach, cliffs, playground, pond

EXPOSURE Mostly shady; less so in winter

TRAFFIC Light–medium; busy on warm-weather weekends and holidays

TRAIL SURFACE Chiefly dirt or sand; some gravel, boardwalk

HIKING TIME 2 hours (with time to hunt for fossils)

DRIVING DISTANCE 56 miles

SEASON Year-round but best from fall to spring

ACCESS Open daily, sunrise–sunset

WHEELCHAIR TRAVERSABLE No

MAPS Maryland Department of Natural Resources, tinyurl.com/calvertcliffsmap

FACILITIES Restrooms at trailhead; portable toilet at beach entrance

CONTACT Maryland Department of Natural Resources, 301-743-7613, tinyurl.com/calvertcliffssp

LOCATION Lusby, Maryland

COMMENTS This park is a popular place to hike and bring families, especially on warm-weather weekends. There are occasions when it's closed after it reaches a maximum number of visitors. During hunting season, the northern half of the park is open to hunters, so hiking is not advised. If you must hike the northern trails during hunting season, wear bright clothing, make noise, and put an orange vest on your dog.

with water lilies, submerged tree trunks, and reeds. The marshlands provide a thriving habitat for turtles, bullfrogs, ducks, and a number of bird species.

The best collecting occurs after a storm—when the fossil supply is replenished—or during low tide. The public beach at Calvert Cliffs State Park is quite small due to erosion of the cliffs, but it's still safe for wading and beachcombing. From the beach, there's a view of Cove Point, a spit of land that once plagued sailors traveling up the Chesapeake Bay to Baltimore. At the end of that spit is Cove Point Light Station, with the oldest continuously working lighthouse in Maryland. It was built in 1828 and is still operational, albeit via automation. On the property, the keeper's home was restored so visitors can stay there overnight.

A recent, unattractive addition to the beach's landscape is Dominion Resources' offshore natural gas transfer platform. The industrial behemoth doesn't totally ruin the view, but it certainly doesn't enhance it. Fortunately, the hikes within Calvert Cliffs State Park are still lovely and worth experiencing. Also be aware that in late fall, a portion of the park is open to hunters. Avoid the northern trails, where hunting is permitted.

For this hike we stayed on the Red Trail and Service Road, where hunting is prohibited. To begin, park at the entrance, where you'll find restrooms, a playground, and picnic tables. The trailhead is to the right of the pond; look for the sign pointing to the Red Trail. Cross over the pond on the boardwalk and head into the woods.

Calvert Cliffs State Park

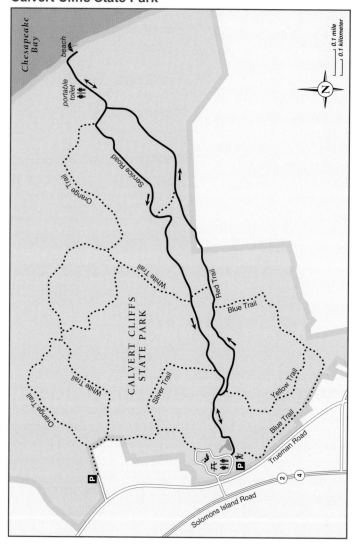

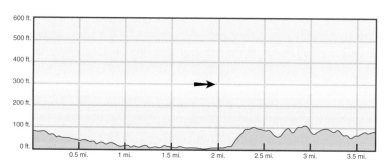

The sand-mulched trail begins in a thick forest with evergreens, deciduous trees, and mature mountain laurel shrubs. The trail is marked with red posts. For a short distance, it joins the service road and then veers right at the first intersection.

Here's where the trail enters the wetlands, crossing boardwalks over moving water as it makes its way to the Chesapeake Bay. Thanks to thick brush and tall trees, it's quite shady and the trail can be wet. The Red Trail intersects with the Yellow Trail, but continue following the red blazes and signs pointing toward the beach. There are some benches that allow you to stop to watch the wildlife frolicking in the wetlands. The hike also has mile markers indicating the distance from the trailhead.

When you get to the swamp, check out all the birds and dragonflies that live there. Listen for the bullfrog mating calls and diving turtles. Other common residents of this magical habitat include wood ducks, great blue herons, lizards, owls, beavers, and snakes. Enjoy watching the busy flights of the birds.

As you cross over the wetlands on the boardwalk, you'll have a breathtaking view of this huge swamp. Yet in the midst of bountiful nature, you may hear a military jet passing overhead from the nearby Patuxent Naval Air Base. When you cross the service road again, you're about 0.2 mile from the beach. Continue straight on the Red Trail as it passes portable toilets. Very soon you'll catch your first glimpse of the beach.

At the opening of the trail, the Chesapeake Bay spreads wide in front of you. There are picnic tables, information about fossil collecting, and a wooden box of toys people have left here for kids. As mentioned earlier, the natural gas platform has obscured what was once a breathtaking vista. However, you can still find lots of shells and hunt for fossils. In the distance is Cove Point Lighthouse. You will probably see a few ships coming down the channel. To the left are Scientist Cliffs, hiding the off-limits nuclear power plant.

Return the way you came, but this time go right at the first intersection, and walk up the hill. This is the service road, consisting of gravel and dirt. You can take the Orange Trail back to the parking lot, although that's not advisable during hunting season. The service road mostly parallels the Red Trail but offers a bit more elevation than the Red Trail for a minor cardio workout.

The road passes through a forest, away from the wetlands and swamp, which is nice during buggy times of year. As you're walking along, you'll pass several intersections. Two point back to the more scenic Red Trail. At the third intersection with the Red Trail, take a left and walk down the hill. After passing a sign for the Yellow Trail, turn right, following the signs to the parking lot.

NEARBY/RELATED ACTIVITIES

Drive south from Calvert Cliffs to visit the charming fishing village of Solomon's Island. Here you'll find several outstanding seafood and crab restaurants, artsy shops, and a boardwalk. Go north for a nearby hike in Flag Ponds Nature Park (410-586-1477, calvertparks.org), where the wide beaches are open to visitors (this park can get very busy in the summer). Battle Creek Cypress Swamp Sanctuary (410-535-5327, calvertparks.org), home to one of the northernmost naturally occurring stands of bald cypress trees in America, is a must-see ecological wonder. Annmarie Sculpture Garden (410-326-4640, annmariegarden.org) is a first-class art museum that both parents and kids love; it's surrounded by a mile-long walking trail with multiple outdoor sculptures.

• •

GPS TRAILHEAD COORDINATES N38° 23.685' W76° 26.108'

> **DIRECTIONS** From the Capital Beltway (I-495) near Forestville, Maryland, take Exit 11A MD 4/Penn Avenue toward Upper Marlboro. Heading south on MD 4, proceed 45 miles to MD 2/MD 4 South to Solomon's Island Road. After 13 miles, turn left into the entrance of Calvert Cliffs State Park.

Calvert Cliffs State Park has acres of thriving wetlands and borders the Chesapeake Bay.

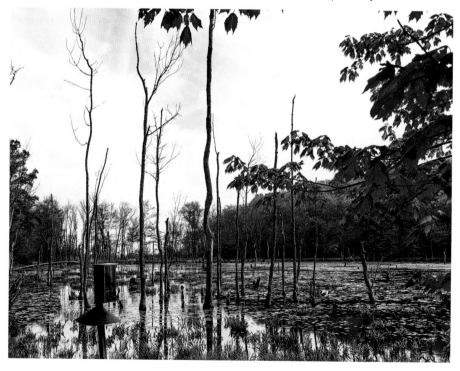

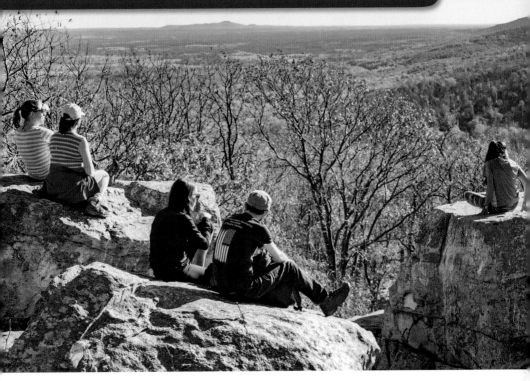

Hikers enjoy the view from Chimney Rock, one of several scenic overlooks at Catoctin Mountain Park.

THIS NATIONAL PARK north of Frederick in Maryland's Blue Ridge region is endowed with a touch of wilderness, a sense of history, and exceptional vistas.

DESCRIPTION

Located scarcely 60 miles northwest of Washington, Catoctin Mountain Park lets arriving visitors know immediately that they are far removed from the urban plains. The air is fresher and cooler, the sky is bigger, trees are everywhere, and the endless ridges rolling softly to the horizon evoke a sense of being in a mountain fastness. As alluring as it is, the area is still recovering from severe despoliation. During the 19th century, Catoctin Mountain—an outlier in the eastern part of the Blue Ridge region— was stripped of timber chiefly for making charcoal for local iron-smelting furnaces. Huge amounts of wood were needed. For instance, making charcoal for 25 years just for the Catoctin Furnace (now a ruin in the state park) required all of the timber on an area much larger than that now covered by the park and the neighboring state park combined. By 1900, much of the Thurmont area had been reduced to logged-over woodlots and submarginal farmlands. Three decades later, the federal government assembled more than 10,500 acres of land as a demonstration project—one of

LENGTH 6.7 miles (with shorter and longer options)

CONFIGURATION Modified loop

DIFFICULTY Moderate

SCENERY Wooded uplands, rock formations, sweeping vistas from overlooks

EXPOSURE Mostly shady; less so in winter

TRAFFIC Light; heavier on warm-weather weekends and holidays; heaviest during fall

TRAIL SURFACE Dirt, sand, rocks

HIKING TIME 4.5–5 hours

DRIVING DISTANCE 60 miles

SEASON Year-round, but best in spring and fall on a clear day so you can appreciate the views

ACCESS Open daily, sunrise–sunset

WHEELCHAIR TRAVERSABLE No

MAPS National Park Service, tinyurl.com/cmptrailmap

FACILITIES Restrooms, water, phone at visitor center and park headquarters

CONTACT 301-663-9388, nps.gov/cato

LOCATION Thurmont, Maryland

COMMENTS This hike combines trails to include four scenic vistas. Each trail is accessible on its own. Many shorter or longer options are available. Avoid hiking here after rainy weather, when the trail is slippery and dangerous. The park is adjacent to Cunningham Falls State Park (page 204), which offers additional recreational opportunities, including a short walk to one of the region's highest and loveliest waterfalls.

about 50 nationally—for restoring the environment and creating recreation facilities. In 1945 the demo area was transferred to the National Park Service (NPS). Nine years later, it was divided roughly in half, with Maryland getting the southern portion for a state park and NPS retaining the rest as Catoctin Mountain Park.

This 6.7-mile hike has a cumulative elevation change of about 1,355 feet. Try the hike in any season, but note that Catoctin's Park Central Road is closed December–March. That road is also closed at times because the park contains the out-of-sight presidential retreat known as Camp David (which began as Franklin D. Roosevelt's Shangri-La). You'll find that the trails are generally kept in good working order and are well signed.

To get started from the visitor center, cross the parking lot to the east; at the trailhead signpost, take the steps to the left, following the signs toward Wolf Rock. The hike starts with an uphill climb and continues with varied terrain winding through the forest among maples, oaks, and dogwoods. At the 0.4-mile marker, where the trail splits, walk straight toward the Thurmont Vista. At the next intersection, continue straight, following the signs to Hog Rock. This part of the trail is a bit rocky and goes sharply downhill for a jaunt and then back uphill. At the top of the hill, turn right to visit the Blue Ridge Summit Overlook. After taking in the view, return to the trail, turn left, and retrace your steps 0.7 mile back toward the Thurmont Vista. When you return to the four-way intersection and a signpost, turn left to follow the 0.5-mile connection to the Thurmont Vista. This part of the trail is mostly gravel and an easy walk. Enjoy the panoramic views of the town of Thurmont, and then continue south for about 0.75 mile, following a wooded ridgeline that's initially level but

Catoctin Mountain Park

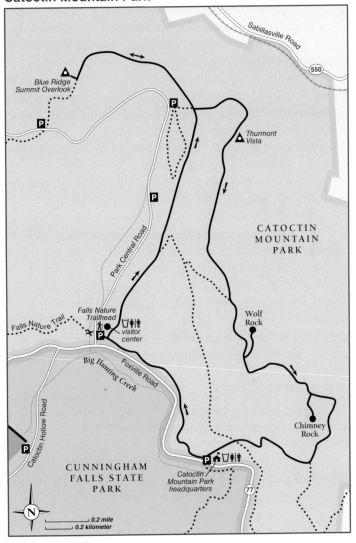

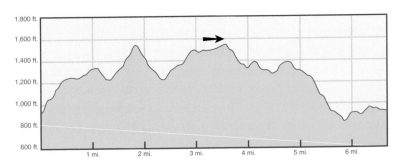

then descends. At a junction, stay left. At the next junction, turn left onto a short side trail leading to Wolf Rock. The quartzite rock formation is a geological wonder that includes a small group of rocks at the far end that forms what looks like the head of a wolf. The quartzite was deposited as layers of sand about 550 million years ago. Covered by other sediments, the quartzite formed when layers of sand were compressed and crystallized during the uplifting of the Appalachian Mountains. Since then, the overlying softer rocks have eroded away, exposing the quartzite. Be careful if you climb the rocks; there are many deep crevices.

Back on the main trail, head for the next overlook, Chimney Rock, 0.5 mile southeast. A right turn onto a short and rocky side trail leads to Chimney Rock, with its big boulders, deep crevices, and glorious views. After visiting the overlook, return to the main trail, keeping right and west as the trail pitches sharply downhill through an understory of mountain laurel. At a four-way intersection, go straight, continuing to descend, near the park headquarters. When you reach MD 77, turn right and follow the trail back to the visitor center. The final mile of the hike has orange and white blazes and parallels the road.

The Wolf Rock/Chimney Rock Loop is the most popular in the park and can be accessed from three places: from the Catoctin Mountain Visitor Center (as described above), from the parking lot in front of the NPS headquarters along MD 77, and from the parking lot on Park Central Road. See a trail map for details. Parking is also available near the Blue Ridge Summit Vista.

NEARBY/RELATED ACTIVITIES

The park offers 25 miles of hiking trails, trout fishing, camping, horseback riding, rock climbing, and cross-country skiing. Visit Cunningham Falls State Park (301-271-7574, tinyurl.com/cunfallspark) to see the waterfall and, in summer, swim in Hunting Creek Lake (page 204). In summer or fall, stop in Thurmont to buy peaches at Pryor's Orchard (301-271-2693, pryorsorchards.com). In mid-October, attend Thurmont's Catoctin Colorfest arts-and-crafts show (colorfest.org).

* *

GPS TRAILHEAD COORDINATES N39° 38.022' W77° 26.963'

DIRECTIONS From the Capital Beltway (I-495), take I-270 north about 32 miles to Frederick. Turn right onto US 15 North (Catoctin Mountain Highway), and proceed about 17 miles to Thurmont. Take the MD 77 exit ramp (on right), turn right at the bottom of the ramp, and proceed west on MD 77 (Foxville Road) about 3 miles. Turn right onto Park Central Road and into Catoctin Mountain Park. Immediately turn right into the visitor center parking lot, or use the overflow parking lot on the left.

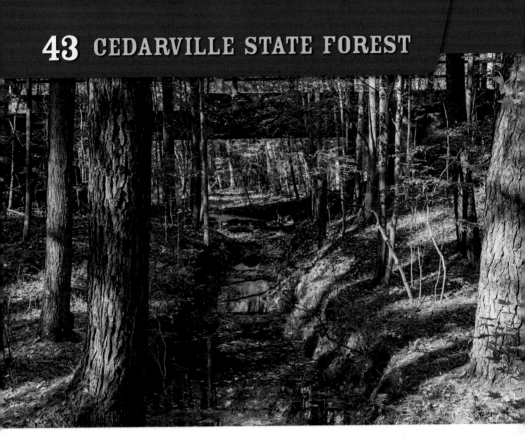

The state forest offers miles of wooded hiking trails and endless wildlife-viewing opportunities.

THE PARK HAS 19.5 MILES of marked trails that wander through the quiet forests of Prince George's and Charles Counties, past pine plantations planted by the Civilian Conservation Corps in the 1930s. The Holly Trail wanders through wooded paths along marshy areas lined with holly, magnolia, and other plants and flowers. The trail is well marked; follow the orange signposts and blazes.

DESCRIPTION

Cedarville State Forest is home to the headwaters of the largest freshwater swamp in Maryland, the Zekiah Swamp, which extends through Charles County for 20 miles and empties into the Wicomico River. The swamp is 1 mile wide and serves as a haven for wildlife. The forest is also home to more than 50 species of trees, including maples, oaks, sweetgums, poplars, hollies, and Virginia pines, attracting a wide variety of birds. In 1930, the Maryland Department of Natural Resources' Forest, Park, and Wildlife Service purchased 2,631 acres of land for a forest demonstration area. Later, 879 more acres were added to bring the total to 3,510 acres.

Begin the hike from the trailhead located in the parking lot next to the information station by the main entrance to the park. The dirt path immediately enters the

LENGTH 6.4 miles (with shorter options)

CONFIGURATION Loop

DIFFICULTY Easy–moderate

SCENERY Woodlands, swamps, streams

EXPOSURE Mostly shady; less so in winter

TRAFFIC Light

TRAIL SURFACE Dirt, sand, gravel

HIKING TIME 3.25–3.5 hours

DRIVING DISTANCE 30 miles

SEASON Year-round

ACCESS Sunrise–sunset. A $3-per-car service charge is payable by the honor system.

WHEELCHAIR TRAVERSABLE No

MAPS Maryland Department of Natural Resources (trail guide available for $3 at park office)

FACILITIES Portable toilet at trailhead parking lot

CONTACT; Maryland Department of Natural Resources, 800-830-3974, tinyurl.com /cedarvillestateforest

LOCATION Brandywine, Maryland

COMMENTS The trail is relatively flat, but you should wear appropriate footwear, as it is often muddy. The Holly Trail is the longest in the park. Shorter hiking options are available, with routes that are 2–4 miles. All trails are shared by hikers, bikers, and equestrians. Watch out for horse manure.

woods. After 0.2 mile the path connects to the Holly Trail, a nearly 7-mile loop that is open for hiking, biking, and horseback riding. Turn left and follow the orange signposts throughout the rest of the hike. The trail includes a lot of twists and turns but is well marked and mostly easy to follow.

When you cross Hidden Springs Road, take the dirt trail to the right as it parallels the road and then diverts back into the forest. After the first mile, when the trail intersects with the white trail, walk left to continue on the orange trail. At the next intersection, turn right as three trails (white, blue, and orange) merge until you reach Sunset Road. Turn left and walk along the gravel fire road. Cross another gravel road and pick up the orange trail again. Now you will start to see orange blazes on the trees. At the next intersection, turn right; you will pass the campground on the left. As you continue on the trail, an empty campsite on the left is a good spot for a picnic. After walking past the campgrounds and the access road, turn right onto the dirt trail. When you come to another gravel road, turn right and you will walk over a boardwalk in front of a small pond with a large beaver dam. The pond is stocked with bluegill, catfish, sunfish, and bass. It is open for bank fishing only (Maryland nontidal license required). Continue through the woods and cross Bee Oak Road three times as it winds back toward your starting point. Just after you pass the 6.5-mile marker, turn left to return to the trailhead. You will know that you went the right way when you see the 6.75-mile marker.

NEARBY/RELATED ACTIVITIES

The nearby towns of Brandywine and Waldorf offer plenty of dining options and shopping destinations.

Cedarville State Forest

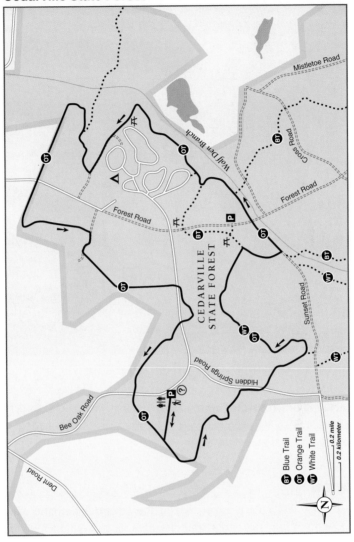

GPS TRAILHEAD COORDINATES N38° 38.817' W76° 49.818'

DIRECTIONS From the Capital Beltway (I-495), take Exit 7A/Branch Avenue (MD 5 South) toward Waldorf. Follow MD 5 for 11.6 miles, and turn left on Cedarville Road. Turn right to stay on Cedarville Road and then right on Bee Oak Road. Drive 1 mile. The parking lot is on the right.

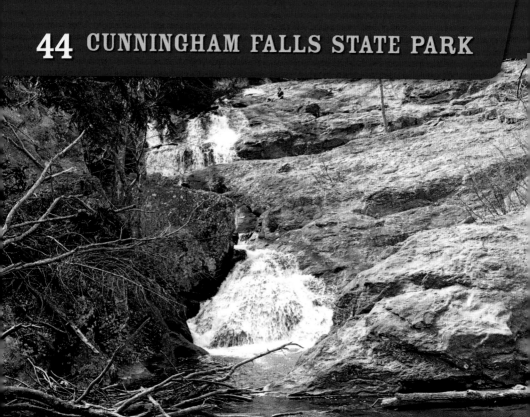

The rushing falls are a scenic attraction and a fun place to visit year-round.

LOCATED NEAR THURMONT, MARYLAND, Cunningham Falls features a beautiful 78-foot cascading waterfall, the largest cascading waterfall in the state, attracting visitors from around the region.

DESCRIPTION

Cunningham Falls State Park is situated in the beautiful Catoctin Mountains in Frederick County. While the parks' trail distances range from 0.5 mile to 7.5 miles, the shortest hike is the most popular, as it leads to the overlook of the cascading waterfalls. The park is divided into two areas: The William Houck Area (3 miles west of Thurmont on MD 77) has the falls and Hunting Creek Lake, and the Manor Area (off of US 15, 3 miles south of Thurmont) is home to the aviary and historic Catoctin Iron Furnace. Both areas have campgrounds. Cunningham Falls lies adjacent to the federally operated Catoctin Mountain Park, which makes the division between the park areas a bit confusing. Together, these three recreation areas offer dozens of miles of hiking trails and an ideal destination for swimming, boating, fishing, picnicking, camping, horseback riding, rock climbing, and cross-country skiing. Campsites and camper cabins are available for rent April–October.

· ·

GPS TRAILHEAD COORDINATES

LOWER FALLS TRAILHEAD: N39° 37.659' W77° 27.830'

FALLS NATURE TRAILHEAD: N39° 38.048' W77° 27.029'

DIRECTIONS From the junction of the Capital Beltway (I-495) and I-270 spur in Maryland, drive northwest on I-270 about 32 miles to Frederick. Take US 15 North (Catoctin Mountain Highway), and proceed about 17 miles to Thurmont. There, take the MD 77 exit ramp (on the right), turn right at the bottom of the ramp, and proceed west on MD 77 (Foxville Road). Turn left into the park at Catoctin Hollow Road.

The boardwalk accessible from MD 77 provides handicap access to the beautiful waterfall.

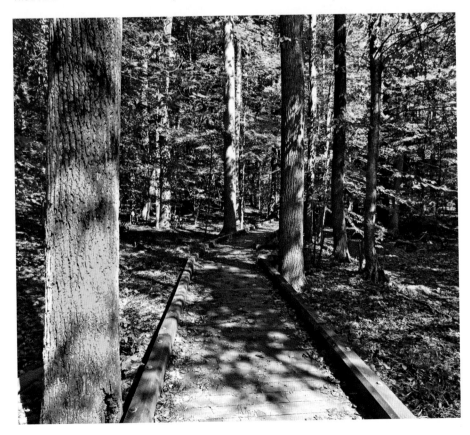

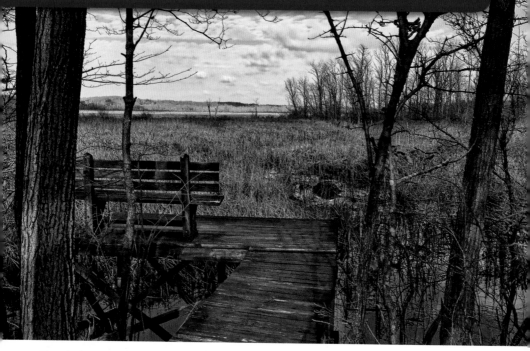

The marshes around Jug Bay are full of wildlife in every season. There are two observation huts and many benches where you can watch the action.

PLANTS AND WILDLIFE THRIVE in the scenic Jug Bay portion of Patuxent River Park in Anne Arundel County. Well-marked trails and observation structures designed for contemplation make this a peaceful and immersive nature experience.

DESCRIPTION

The Patuxent River, Maryland's longest in-state waterway, wriggles south more than 100 miles through woodlands, wetlands, farmlands, and urbanized areas to reach Chesapeake Bay. Like the rest of the bay's watershed, it suffers from poor water quality. In 1985, however, the river valley became part of the Chesapeake Bay National Estuarine Research Reserve Maryland, which promotes coastal research and conducts system-wide monitoring of water-quality and nutrient data. The reserve consists of more than 6,000 acres of salt marshes that provide habitat for herons, egrets, and striped bass.

Named for a lakelike stretch of the river, Jug Bay is also supported by Friends of Jug Bay, volunteers who provide critical support to the preserve with education, fundraising, and research projects, including daily monitoring of the water quality from Jug Bay's Railroad Bed Trail. The Jug Bay Wetlands Sanctuary spearheads staff-led

LENGTH 3 miles (with longer option)

CONFIGURATION Modified loop

DIFFICULTY Easy–moderate

SCENERY Meadows, tidal marshes, river views, hilly woodlands

EXPOSURE Shady; less so in winter

TRAFFIC Usually very light–light; heavier on warm-weather weekends and holidays, near visitor center, and in nature study area

TRAIL SURFACE Mostly hard-packed sand; some pavement; short stretches of board-walk, wood chips, mud

HIKING TIME 1.5 hours (with time for observation)

DRIVING DISTANCE 23 miles

ACCESS Open Wednesdays, Fridays, and Saturdays, 8 a.m.–5 p.m.; day-use fee: $6 per person

WHEELCHAIR TRAVERSABLE In some places

MAPS Free sketch map available at visitor center; tinyurl.com/jugbaytrailmap

FACILITIES Water, restrooms, and phone at visitor center; picnic tables

CONTACT 410-741-9330, jugbay.org

LOCATION Lothian, Maryland

COMMENTS Dogs are not permitted. Hunting is allowed, so check the Jug Bay website calendar, or call the park office before you go. The National Audubon Society named Jug Bay a Nationally Important Bird Area, so take along field glasses and reference books.

environmental-education programs, and families can learn a great deal about the landscape by touring the kid-friendly visitor center. The McCann Wetlands Center is an interactive museum and meeting space, with picnic areas and an observation deck. There's a small pen with goats wearing coats (in winter) on the property.

The 8 miles of hiking trails wind their way through several areas of great natural beauty dotted along the lower Patuxent. Jug Bay scenery consists of vistas, trails, beaver and crab habitats, and birds. Most visitors focus on attractions rather than hiking. They'll spend time at the visitor center, River Farm, Community Garden, and Glendening Nature Preserve with its restored Plummer Farmhouse. Together, these areas form one of the finest mid-Atlantic birding spots.

The drive to Jug Bay is on a dirt road through a forest past ANIMALS CROSSING signs alerting you to watch for turtles. After the leaves fall off the trees, you can see Jug Bay to your right as you enter the park. The sanctuary is open only on Wednesdays, Fridays, and Saturdays, with an occasional Sunday event.

At the McCann Wetlands Center, there is a picnic pavilion and ample parking. Inside the Wetlands Center is a small interactive museum with educational activities for children, restrooms, and a small shop. The museum explains that these wetlands are home to reptiles such as the eastern box turtle, black rat snake, fence lizard, garter snake, worm snake, hognose snake, spotted turtle, northern water snake, red-bellied turtle, eastern painted turtle, and common musk turtle. Snapping turtles, salamanders, tree frogs, toads, wood frogs, spring peepers, bullfrogs, pickerel frogs, and southern leopard frogs also make their home in the marshes here.

Jug Bay Wetlands Sanctuary

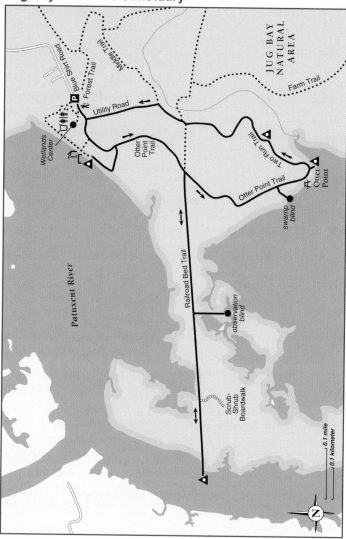

Visit the expansive observation deck in front of the McCann Wetlands Center. To the left of the deck you'll see a sign pointing to the Otter Point Trailhead. Begin following this trail, and soon you'll come to a detour pointing down some stairs to a boardwalk over the marshes. The boardwalk ascends to the creek bank to reach level ground. Follow the boardwalk along the shoreline to a wooden bench. Here you can look out at a few houses in the distance and hear the waves lapping against the shore. It's a beautiful perspective and worth the short climb back up the hill to return to the Otter Point Trail.

Turn right at the intersection and continue into the forest, following the Otter Point Trail. There are signposts along this trail with a QR code. Scan the code using an app on your smartphone to learn specific details about the wetlands.

At the next intersection, turn right to follow the Railroad Bed Trail, a rail-to-trail path over a spit of land that cuts across the wetlands. The trail passes between Upper and Lower Glebe Marshes north of Jug Bay. About halfway across, you'll come to a boardwalk protruding through the scrub marshes into Jug Bay. The observation blind is an ideal place to find some shade and watch the birds without scaring them away. As you walk to the blind, check out this shallow tidal pool where turtles, frogs, and snakes find the nutrients and coverage they need to survive.

Return to the Railroad Bed Trail, turn left, and continue walking toward the end of the spit. Make another brief detour onto the Scrub-Shrub Boardwalk to learn more about this marsh plant that sustains and filters the water from Jug Bay and the Patuxent River. In the warm-weather months, it's filled with cattails, other aquatic plants, and noisy amphibians.

As you get closer to the end of the trail, you'll see a mansion on the bluff to the right. This Federal-style home is part of the Mount Calvert Historical and Archaeological Park. This park in Upper Marlboro interprets the history of the American Indians; Charles Town, Prince George's county seat; and the African American heritage of Mount Calvert Plantation.

Surprisingly, the spit ends before reaching the other side of the bay. At its terminus, you'll find canoe storage and a metal platform called the Jug Bay River Pier. Equipment on the pier is used to monitor the water quality of Jug Bay and the Patuxent River. Turn back, retracing your steps to the intersection of the Otter Point Trail. Turn right, going past the swamp blind and out to the trail's namesake, Otter Point, where there is a large stand of holly trees, a picnic table, and a bench. There's also a small dock with another bench where you can observe Jug Bay and Beaver Pond, a habitat for crabs and beavers.

On your way back from Otter Point, turn right to join the Two Run Trail, following the white blazes. This trail skirts the shoreline and continues through the forest. To your right will be the swampy Beaver Pond, where the beavers have chewed their way through countless tree trunks. There's another observation deck here.

Continue following the white blazes up a hill. Check out signs identifying the unique collection of trees in this forest (such as the persimmon). When you get to the intersection of the Two Run Trail and Railroad Bed Trail, turn right toward Two Run and the wetlands center. Walk down the wooden steps. On your right you'll see a small bridge leading to the Upper Railroad Bed Trail. If you have time, you can take that trail to River Farm Point. Otherwise, return to the wetlands center and the parking lot.

NEARBY/RELATED ACTIVITIES

The Patuxent Rural Life Museums (301-627-6074, tinyurl.com/patuxmuseums) are generally open April–October on Saturdays and Sunday afternoons. They include a tool museum, a blacksmith shop, a tobacco farming museum, and an 1880s log cabin. In the warm-weather months, sign up for a guided birding walk, nature hike, or river ecology boat tour there, or take a rental canoe or kayak out on the bay.

If you have time, roam at least some of the adjoining 1,670-acre Merkle Wildlife Sanctuary (entrance fee; in winter, it's open weekends only, 10 a.m.–4 p.m.; after May 1, it's open daily, 10 a.m.–5 p.m.) and any of its four hiking trails. Be sure to visit the observation platform, which is a fine spot for bird sightings. Also stop by the Frank Oslislo Visitor Center. For information and directions, call 301-888-1410 or visit tinyurl.com/merklews.

• •

GPS TRAILHEAD COORDINATES N38° 47.092' W76° 42.048'

> **DIRECTIONS** From the Capital Beltway (I-495) near Forestville, Maryland, take Exit 11A heading southeast on MD 4 for 23 miles. Take a right on Plummer Lane, and then another right on Wrighton Road. Turn left at the sign pointing to Jug Bay Wetlands Sanctuary, past Blue Shirt Road. Then enter the parking lot near the visitor center and park office.

Jug Bay Visitor Center has interesting exhibits on ecology and the region's wetland environment.

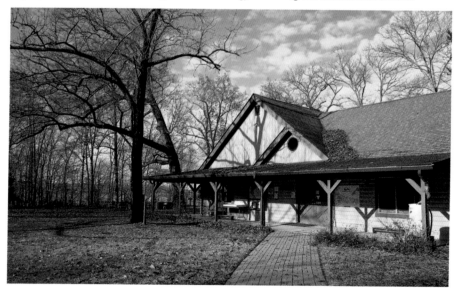

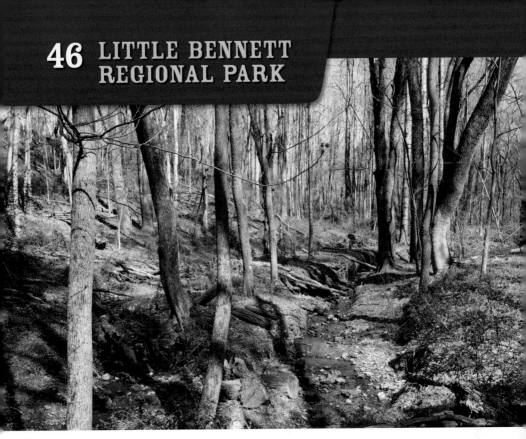

This regional park offers miles of hiking trails to explore in a quiet setting.

AT 3,700 ACRES, Little Bennett Regional Park is the largest in Montgomery County and offers more than 21 miles of natural-surface trails, along with hiking, camping, golfing, and equestrian opportunities.

DESCRIPTION

Located in Montgomery County's most rural area, bordering Frederick County, the park is mostly forested and lies among the tributaries of Little Bennett Creek. The terrain ranges from easy wooded sections to steep hills to open meadows, with an abundance of native plants.

Park at the Kingsley parking area, and begin your hike on the Hard Cider Trail. The trailhead is on the left. The beginning tends to be muddy, so be prepared and careful as you begin your walk. The trail is accessible to horses, so you are also likely to encounter manure along the way.

Follow this trail for a mile, and cross a footbridge. Turn left uphill on the Purdum Trail, and in a short distance the trail will split. Take the left fork and continue to where the trail joins a gravel service road. Stay left on the service road until you reach the hike-in campground. There is a portable toilet on the right and a large fire ring with

LENGTH 6.2 miles (with shorter and longer options)

CONFIGURATION Loop with many trail changes

DIFFICULTY Moderate

SCENERY Wooded hills, meadow vistas, stream valleys

EXPOSURE Shady; less so in winter

TRAFFIC Usually very light

TRAIL SURFACE Mostly dirt, plus some gravel, grass, and pine needles; rocky, rooty, and muddy in places

HIKING TIME 3.5–4 hours

DRIVING DISTANCE 40 miles

SEASON Year-round

ACCESS Open daily, sunrise–sunset; no entry fee. The park is also easily accessible from I-270 and just north of the more developed communities of Clarksburg and Germantown.

Campground is open April–November; 91 wooded campsites are available.

WHEELCHAIR TRAVERSABLE No

MAPS Montgomery Parks, littlebennettcampground.com

FACILITIES None at trailhead; phone at Hawk's Reach Activity Center; roadside restrooms, water, and phone near campground's loop C; portable toilet on Purdum Trail

CONTACT 301-528-3430

LOCATION Clarksburg, Maryland

COMMENTS The park has numerous relatively short trails that connect so that you can create a loop hike of varying lengths. Most are well marked and maintained, but we highly recommend using a trail map or GPS. Maps are available at the information stands at all trailheads. The trails north of Hyattstown Mill Road are shared by hikers, equestrians, and cyclists, while the ones south of Hyattstown Mill Road are for hiking only.

picnic tables on the left. Continue straight to the intersection of Browning Run Trail. Turn left. Follow the trail downhill, and cross a creek and wooden walkway.

After you cross the walkway, the trail enters a field. Stay right and continue to the top of the rise to the intersection of the Pine Knob Trail. Turn right, downhill, on the Tobacco Barn Trail, passing another field on the left. The Tobacco Barn Trail will then cross Browning Run. There is no footbridge at this crossing, so you will have to straddle some rocks to cross the stream.

The Tobacco Barn Trail will climb through another field and pass an unofficial trail on the left; it then arrives at the ridge, where you will see the ruins of a farm site from the late 19th century. Continue straight on the Timber Ridge Trail. Pass another unofficial trail on the right where the Timber Ridge Trail turns left. You'll be walking along a steep ridgeline on the side of the hill with great views of the forest to the left. Look for the wooden walkway, and continue to where the Timber Ridge Trail ends at the intersection of the Pine Grove Trail. Turn left.

Follow the trail to the Western Piedmont Trail. Stay left on the gravel service road/Western Piedmont Trail, and pass the small Earls' Picnic Ground. Follow the Western Piedmont Trail for the remainder of the hike. You will pass bluebird-nest boxes and information displays that give details about the wetland plants and wildlife in the park. Learn about critters such as spotted turtles, spotted salamanders,

Little Bennett Regional Park

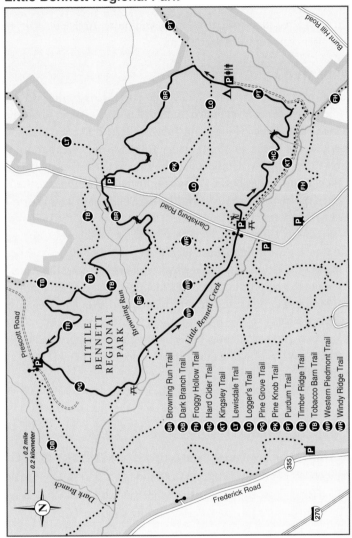

BR Browning Run Trail
DB Dark Branch Trail
FH Froggy Hollow Trail
HC Hard Cider Trail
KT Kingsley Trail
LT Lewisdale Trail
LO Logger's Trail
PG Pine Grove Trail
PK Pine Knob Trail
PT Purdum Trail
TR Timber Ridge Trail
TB Tobacco Barn Trail
WP Western Piedmont Trail
WR Windy Ridge Trail

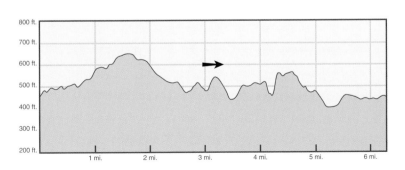

red-spotted newts, woodcocks, barred owls, and more. Arrive back at the Kingsley parking area after crossing Clarksburg Road.

NEARBY/RELATED ACTIVITIES

The park offers many combinations of trails, allowing for longer or shorter hikes. For a 3-mile sampler, drive along Hyattstown Mill Road to Earl's Picnic Area, and do a loop using the Pine Grove, Timber Ridge, and Tobacco Barn Trails, and then the road.

The park is also home to Montgomery County's only campground and Little Bennett Golf Course but is significant for housing several historic sites: the Montgomery Chapel Cemetery (a burial ground for former parishioners), the Zeigler Log House (a mid-19th-century home), Hyattstown Mill (a saw- and gristmill from the 1790s to 1930s), Hyattstown Miller's House (the residence of the miller until 1930s), the Perry Browning House (an 18th-century farm and house; not open to the public), the Charles Browning House (a 19th-century farmhouse), Kings Distillery (the former site of a 19th-century rye whiskey distillery), and the Kingsley School House. The schoolhouse is one of the few 19th-century one-room schoolhouses that still exist in Montgomery County. It is furnished and maintained as it would have looked in the late 1920s.

Hawk's Reach Activity Center at Little Bennett Campground (301-528-3430, montgomeryparks.org) offers guided hikes, activities, nature films, and other special events.

• •

GPS TRAILHEAD COORDINATES N39° 15.956' W77° 16.803'

> **DIRECTIONS** From the Capital Beltway (I-495), take I-270 North. At Exit 18, go right on MD 121 (Clarksburg Road). Continue on Clarksburg Road across MD 355 (Frederick Road). Enter Little Bennett Regional Park and turn right into the third parking lot, the Kingsley parking area.

47 MAGRUDER BRANCH TRAIL AND LOWER MAGRUDER TRAIL

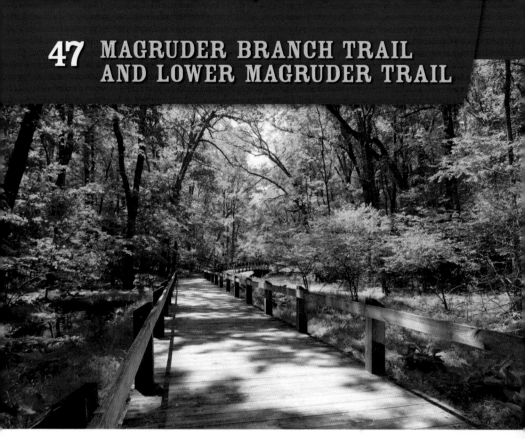

MacGruder Branch offers a shady oasis in which to enjoy a leisurely walk or run.

DAMASCUS RECREATIONAL PARK is 284 acres and has multiple outdoor athletic fields and courts for general recreation opportunities. A stream valley that runs adjacent to the park has a modest trail system that enables hikers in the northernmost part of Montgomery County to enjoy a restful woodland setting where plants and animals thrive.

DESCRIPTION

This out-and-back hike can be extended to 7.3 miles one-way. It starts with part of a paved trail that extends north to Damascus. It then continues on a dirt trail that extends south to Seneca Creek.

Start your hike from the parking-lot trailhead at Damascus Regional Park and proceed uphill on the paved Magruder Branch Trail. As you begin the hike, you will pass tennis courts, a picnic shelter, a playground, and a ballfield. After you pass some sheds and additional parking, continue straight to head north and stay on Magruder Branch Trail. To the right, Lower Magruder Branch begins and extends to the south. As you continue straight ahead, the trail becomes wooded and shady. Cross over a bridge and a stream, and follow the trail as it turns left. The trail alternates between asphalt and

LENGTH 6.4 miles (with shorter and longer options)

CONFIGURATION Out-and-back

DIFFICULTY Easy

SCENERY Parklands, woodlands, stream valleys

EXPOSURE Mostly shady; less so in winter

TRAFFIC Very light–light; heaviest in vicinity of sports facilities on warm-weather weekends and holidays

TRAIL SURFACE Asphalt and boardwalk

HIKING TIME 2.5–3 hours

DRIVING DISTANCE 40 miles

SEASON Year-round

ACCESS Open daily, sunrise–sunset. Various

trail connectors feed into the park from neighborhood streets. Parking lots along the trail are located at Damascus Regional Park, Valley Park Drive, and Log House Road.

WHEELCHAIR TRAVERSABLE No

MAPS Montgomery Parks, tinyurl.com/magrudertrails

FACILITIES Restrooms and water at shelter close to trailhead

CONTACT Montgomery Parks, montgomeryparks.org

LOCATION Damascus, Maryland

COMMENTS Watch for poison ivy. The trail has been under construction for several years. Equipment may be parked along the trail, and some of the surface is disrupted. Parallel trails allow the entire trail to be passable.

wooded boardwalk and continues straight several miles. The mostly deciduous trees are the usual local mix of oak, hickory, and beech, plus some conifers. When you come to Sweepstakes Road, make a right, cross the street carefully, and continue on the trail. You can make the hike longer or shorter depending on where you park and how far you feel like walking. You can turn around at any point. It is a popular spot for dog walking and jogging. You will see an occasional bicyclist, but the boardwalks and limited length make this a less-than-ideal bike path.

NEARBY/RELATED ACTIVITIES

Detour to family-owned Butler's Orchard (301-972-3299, butlersorchard.com), which has pick-your-own strawberries, apples, blueberries, pumpkins, and more.

• •

GPS TRAILHEAD COORDINATES N39° 14.651' W77° 13.346'

DIRECTIONS From the junction of the Capital Beltway (I-495) and I-270 spur in Maryland, head northwest on I-270 (toward Frederick) about 15 miles. Get off at Exit 16, and proceed 0.5 mile on the exit ramp, staying right at the fork (marked Exit 16A/Damascus). Merge onto Ridge Road, and proceed 4.3 miles (crossing MD 355). Turn right onto Kings Valley Road; proceed 0.6 mile, turn left into the park's first entrance, and go about 100 yards to the parking lot near the playing field.

Magruder Branch Trail and Lower Magruder Trail

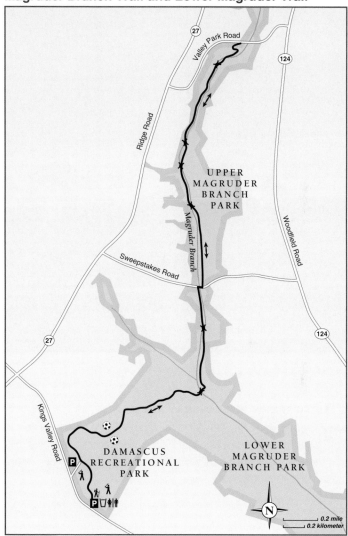

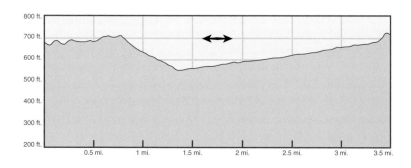

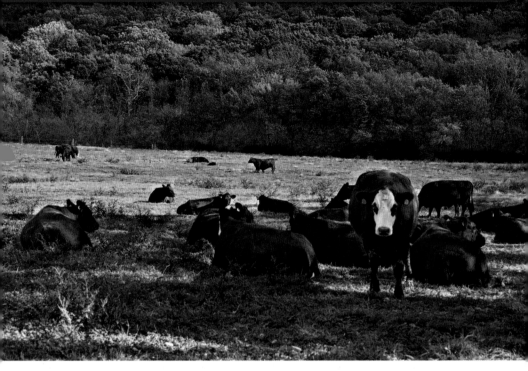

The battlefield includes scenic views of farmland, forested hills, and valleys.

THIS LESSER-KNOWN BUT LOVINGLY PRESERVED Civil War battlefield is operated by the National Park Service. Along with a visitor center, it has multiple hikes in three areas, which require a car to access. The hikes explore the grounds of an old mill and historic farm that straddles the Monocacy (pronounced muh-NOCK-a-see) River.

DESCRIPTION

Begin your visit at the Monocacy National Battlefield Visitor Center, where you can pick up a trail map and learn the significance of this one-day battle. In the summer of 1864, near the end of the Civil War, the South made its last attempt to carry the war north, as Confederate general Jubal Early led his troops from the Shenandoah Valley onto this land near the prosperous town of Frederick. The ultimate goal was to capture Washington, D.C. The Union soldiers, led by Major General Lew Wallace, were outnumbered three to one, and the fierce fight ended with a Confederate victory, despite massive casualties—more than 900 rebels died here. The fight allowed Union troops to send reinforcements to Washington, D.C., which deterred further efforts by the Confederates to invade the nation's capital. The visitor center has a

LENGTH Two hikes: 0.7 mile and 3.5 miles

CONFIGURATION Two separate loops

DIFFICULTY Easy–moderate

SCENERY Forested hills and valleys, farmland, historic landmarks, rocky riverbank

EXPOSURE Partially shady; much less so in winter

TRAFFIC Usually very light

TRAIL SURFACE Mostly dirt or grass

HIKING TIME 2 hours (with time to check out the national battlefield visitor center)

DRIVING DISTANCE 50 miles

SEASON Year-round, but best in fall and spring

ACCESS Open daily, sunrise–sunset. Dogs must be on a leash.

WHEELCHAIR TRAVERSABLE No

MAPS National Park Service, tinyurl.com/monocacymap

FACILITIES Visitor center has restrooms, a gift shop, exhibits, and a scenic viewing area; it also offers self-guided touring and hiking maps.

CONTACT National Park Service, 301-662-3515, nps.gov/mono

LOCATION Frederick, Maryland

COMMENTS This historic battlefield consists of multiple properties and the surrounding farmland.

map showing the movement of the troops and an observation deck where you can see the landscape and imagine how the battle played out.

To begin your hike, drive from the visitor center to Gambrill Mill (stop 5 on the self-guided history tour). The Gambrill Mill trailhead is by the parking lot and begins on a boardwalk built over a creek surrounded by huge trees that were probably here during the fateful battle. Because the slow-moving stream is covered by forest, the first part of this half-mile hike is in the shade. You'll pass some benches where you can sit and contemplate the history of what took place here and read the interpretive signs along the way.

Stop at the overlook, where you can see what had been a covered wooden bridge in 1864 but today is concrete and called the Urbana Pike Bridge. The Confederates sent 15,000 speeding troops with horses, wagons, and artillery toward the battlefield over the original bridge, which of course was burned down afterward. Step off the trail, and walk down the hill to the Monocacy River shoreline. Here you'll have panoramic views of the railroad bridge and the Urbana Pike Bridge crossing over the slow-moving river. It is a beautiful site.

Return to the trail, where the remainder of the loop meanders through a grassy field paralleling the river and picket fence. Up on the hill, at the end of the hike, you'll see Edgewood, the Gambrill family's home, an elaborate Second Empire–style mansion that is now used by the National Park Service as offices. The flour mill is a national historic landmark; it's a regal stone building with picnic tables and a bench where you can sit and enjoy the serenity of the scenery. During the battle, the mill was transformed into a Confederate field hospital.

Monocacy National Battlefield

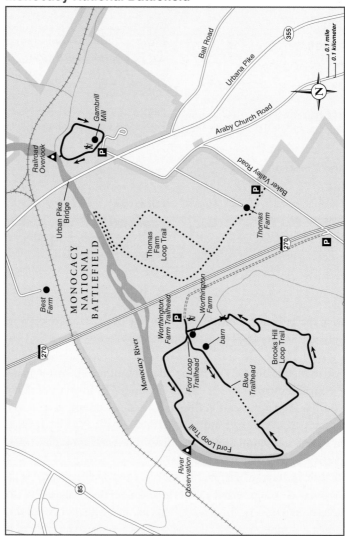

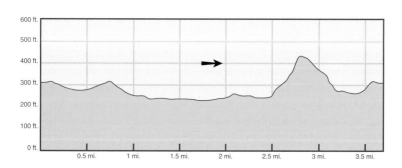

To get to the second part of the hike, drive across VA 355 down Araby Church Road, and then onto Baker Valley Road. Then take the long, gravel road toward Worthington Farm, and park in the lot. The hike starts out on a continuation of the gravel road. You'll walk past the Worthington Farmhouse and the fenced-in meadow of cows. When you see the sign for the blue trail, make a U-turn and begin heading back toward the farmhouse.

Back by the farmhouse, look left for the entrance to the Ford Loop Trail. It begins at the opening in the fence. You'll see a blue-blazed trail leading into the woods; the pasture will be to your left and the riverbank on the right. Follow this narrow dirt trail. It encompasses a section of the battlefield where Confederate forces crossed the Monocacy River onto the grounds of Worthington Farm and prepared to attack the Union troops. John Worthington owned this 300-acre farm, where he grew wheat and corn and had a pasture of fruit trees (the remnants of which you will see on this hike). During the Worthingtons' time here, there were two barns and slave quarters on the property. While the battle raged, the Worthington family hid in the basement. Confederate soldiers took over the home. Today, a rancher leases the meadow, and a herd of black and white cattle graze in it.

At first the trail travels down some uneven log steps as it moves closer to the Ballenger Creek, which empties into the Monocacy River. The rooty trail continues through the woods and is very easy to follow thanks to the clear markings with arrows and blue blazes. The trail makes a right turn, and you'll cross a tiny footbridge and reenter the woods.

At this point, the woods get thicker and Ballenger Creek has widened substantially. You're in a lowland environment ideal for moisture-seeking trees, including sycamore, maple, box elder, and willow. Take a short detour to the shoreline so you can see some of the cottages across the river. Once there, you'll see dozens of empty clamshells. You might hear some toads calling to one another, or see crayfish, salamanders, and even ducks.

The trail continues to skirt the creek, and you have great views of rapids. At this point, the trail moves left and you'll come to a clearing. At the clearing, you'll have an impressive view of Brooks Hill in the distance with foothills of clover. Keep your eyes out for furry varmints.

When you see the intersection of Brooks Hill Loop and the Ford Loop Trail, take a right and begin your ascent of Brooks Hill. If you're not up for the climb, you can follow the gravel farm road back to the farmhouse and parking lot. On Brooks Hill Loop, you'll begin by walking through the edge of a pasture and might get close to a few curious cows. At a grove of withered-looking apple trees, you'll see a sign pointing to the Brooks Loop Trail and reenter the woods. This trail is so lightly used that you will definitely see a lot of wildlife, such as deer and rabbits. The trees in the upland forest are mostly oak and hickory. The abundant nuts from these trees are what attracts so much wildlife.

Next you'll cross a boardwalk and bridge, where you begin climbing the hill. There's very little ground cover here, as the trees are closely spaced. Stay on the trail and enjoy the slow burn in your legs as you follow the blue blazes along the ridge. The effort is worth it for the panoramic view. The trail slowly descends, and you'll pass a small stone wall and giant root ball from a fallen tree. When the hike levels out, you'll cross a dry creekbed over a wooden bridge. At this point, you'll pass through a stand of overgrown fruit trees that are leaning over and look kind of spooky. Just after this grove, you'll be back at the Worthington Farmhouse and the Civil War–era cannon at the end of the trail.

NEARBY/RELATED ACTIVITIES

The battlefield is just a few miles from historic Frederick. Check out Carroll Creek Linear Park (cityoffrederick.com), a walkway along the Monocacy River with shops, restaurants, and special events. Check out the National Museum of Civil War Medicine (301-695-1864, civilwarmed.org). This engrossing museum gives visitors a sense of how difficult it was for doctors to care for the wounded and how little they knew about the dangers of cross contamination. If you're thirsty for a cold beer, the Flying Dog Brewery (301-694-7899, flyingdogbrewery.com) offers the chance to learn how this superb beer is produced and to sample a few at the end.

• •

GPS TRAILHEAD COORDINATES N39° 21.548' W77° 24.350'

> **DIRECTIONS** From the Capital Beltway (I-495) take I-270 North and drive 28 miles. Take Exit 31A and merge onto MD 85 North toward Market Street. Turn right onto Spectrum Drive. Go three-quarters of the way around the traffic circle to the third exit onto Holiday Drive. Take a right on MD 355; Monocacy National Battlefield Visitor Center is on the right at 5201 Urbana Park.

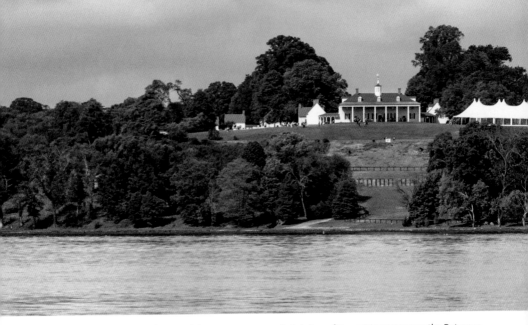

From the National Colonial Farm, visitors can see a wonderful view of Mount Vernon across the Potomac.

PISCATAWAY PARK IS NAMED FOR the Piscataway Creek and its namesake American Indians, who were once one of the most populous tribes in the Chesapeake Bay region. In the late 18th century, the view across the Potomac River from George Washington's Mount Vernon was one of woods and cultivated fields. More than two centuries later, it still is.

DESCRIPTION

In the early 1950s, a mix of private and public actions saved the shoreline across from Mount Vernon from development, with local groups and citizens launching an effort to protect it. Then, in 1961, Congress authorized Piscataway Park to preserve "the historic and scenic values . . . of lands which provide the principal overview." Using more easements than ownership, the present-day park extends along the Potomac River about 6 miles and covers about 5,000 acres.

The Accokeek Foundation, in partnership with the National Park Service, manages about 200 acres within the park at the National Colonial Farm. This hike combines all the trails within the 200-acre historic farm museum. The property demonstrates 18th-century agriculture, including a reconstructed Colonial-era farm

LENGTH 3.4 miles

CONFIGURATION Modified loop

DIFFICULTY Easy–moderate

SCENERY River views, farmland, woodlands, wetlands

EXPOSURE Mostly open; more so in winter

TRAFFIC Very light–light; heavier on warm-weather weekends and holidays

TRAIL SURFACE Chiefly dirt or grass, with marsh boardwalk, short stretches of gravel, and pavement

HIKING TIME 2.5 hours (allow extra time to visit historic farm attractions)

DRIVING DISTANCE 22 miles

ACCESS Open daily, sunrise–sunset. Visitor center is open March 1–November 30, Tuesday–Sunday, 10 a.m.–4 p.m., and December 1–February 28, 10 a.m.–4 p.m., on weekends only.

WHEELCHAIR TRAVERSABLE No

MAPS National Park Service, tinyurl.com /npspiscatawaymap; Accokeek Foundation, tinyurl.com/accokeekfoundmap

FACILITIES Restrooms, water at visitor center (near trailhead; see hours above)

CONTACT Accokeek Foundation at Piscataway, 301-283-2113, accokeekfoundation.org

LOCATION Accokeek, Maryland

COMMENTS Stay on trails and avoid trespassing; although the park is under National Park Service management, much of it is privately owned property on which scenic easements permit limited land use by the public.

featuring now-rare crops and livestock breeds, as well as a modern organic farm. Among its other attractions are views of Mount Vernon, a chestnut grove, an arboretum, and a marsh. The mostly level hike is only partially blazed and signposted. The hand-drawn map available at the visitor center provides a good overview of the site; however, be advised that the trail details are not completely accurate.

To get started, walk out the back door of the visitor center, and visit the fishing pier, as it offers a view of Mount Vernon year-round. Return to the dirt path and head west. Just before getting to the avenue of cedars, turn right and walk across the grass to the signposted Riverview Trail. It's an open, blue-blazed, mowed-in-season grassy trail that's 0.8 mile long but hidden from the river by thickets. On approaching a fenced enclosure, leave the trail to turn right, and then turn right again to take a stairway to another boat dock that provides a closer view of Mount Vernon.

Continuing on the Riverview Trail, detour to the enclosure known as the Museum Garden. A key part of the National Colonial Farm, it features plants grown and used by the colonists. Later you'll see more of the farm and perhaps some staff members and volunteers, who wear period garb and interact informatively with visitors. Back on the main trail, stop at the reconstructed 18th-century tobacco barn, where you can step inside to get a glimpse of drying tobacco. If you enjoy farm animals, take a few minutes to visit with the turkeys and chickens as they waddle around the farmyard.

After leaving the tobacco farm, turn left, walk to the end of the fence, and turn right onto a gravel road. After passing the caretaker's residence, a driveway, and an

National Colonial Farm at Piscataway Park

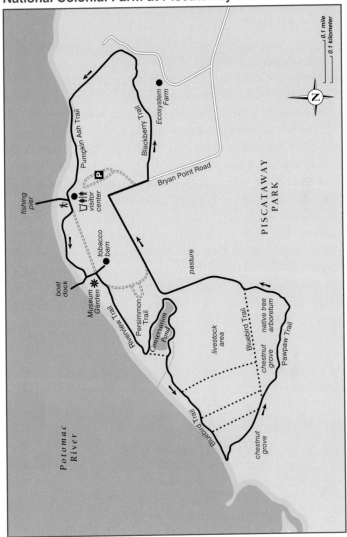

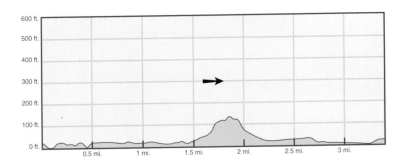

old outkitchen on the right, leave the road and swing right onto a grassy trail (part of the Riverview Trail). After a short distance, turn left onto the Persimmon Trail, and follow it around Conservation Pond. The pond serves as valuable habitat for fish, frogs, turtles, ducks, geese, beavers, and other wildlife.

After following the loop around the pond, swing sharply right and head into the woods on a dirt trail. Soon after crossing a stream and out in the open again, turn right at the first junction, and walk past overgrown fields. Turn right at the next junction. This is now the Bluebird Trail, which contains a handful of nest boxes for eastern bluebirds. Continue onto the signposted and white-blazed Pawpaw Trail, a narrow dirt trail that arcs half a mile through a hilly and heavily wooded area. This is the only trail that has a significant change in elevation. The trail is named for the pawpaw (also spelled papaw) tree, which grows in abundance in the park and produces green oblong fruits.

The Pawpaw Trail ends at the upper edge of a mowed area dotted with trees and shrubs representing more than 125 species that grew in southern Maryland in the Colonial period. They make up the park's 6-acre Native Tree Arboretum, started in the 1980s. Roam among the plants, and then follow the edge of the woods west (away from the Pawpaw Trail). Turn left onto a gravel road (part of the Bluebird Trail), walk 10 yards, and turn left again onto a grassy path to semicircle around what

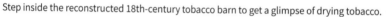

Step inside the reconstructed 18th-century tobacco barn to get a glimpse of drying tobacco.

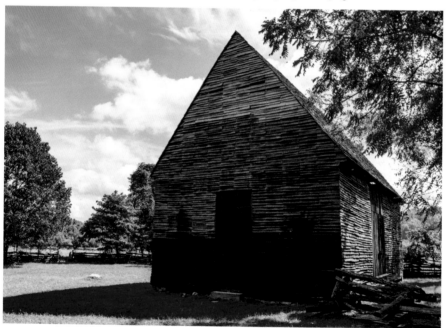

park literature alleges is a chestnut grove. Continuing, you'll arrive at the junction of the Pawpaw Trail and the short trail up from the Bluebird Trail. This time, turn right onto the short trail and then right again onto the blue-blazed Bluebird Trail, and head out into the open.

Follow the road east, between a pasture on the left and the lower part of the arboretum on the right. Beyond the pasture, turn sharply left to stay on the gravel road and Bluebird Trail. Heading north, follow the road as it swings right past the farm's livestock area. The trail ends near a barn that houses red Milking Devon cattle, Ossabaw Island hogs, and Spanish turkeys. Continue on the gravel road past cow pastures, fields of geese, and the original homestead. Turn right onto the paved Bryan Point Road. Pass the first intersection, and walk about 50 yards. Turn left onto the Blackberry Trail at a half-hidden trail sign. Follow the purple blazes through the woods.

At the far side, you'll reach the fenced-in, 8-acre Robert Ware Straus Ecosystem Farm. It develops improved methods of intensive and sustainable organic farming. The signage here is easy to miss, so be sure to note that just before you reach the farm, the Blackberry Trail diverts left and runs along the edge of the woods until it reaches the waterfront. At the next trail junction, proceed on the signposted and yellow-blazed Pumpkin Ash Trail, and cross a wooden boardwalk and marshland that leads back to the visitor center.

NEARBY/RELATED ACTIVITIES

Don't miss a side trip to the half-mile (one-way) Marsh Boardwalk Trail, located just a few miles from the National Colonial Farm at the end of a road that branches off of Bryan Point Road. The habitat, protected by Piscataway Park, provides birders an opportunity to see many types of birds, including ospreys, herons, loons, ducks, bald eagles, and more. Other activities at the park include fishing and boating.

• •

GPS TRAILHEAD COORDINATES N38° 41.724' W77° 03.956'

DIRECTIONS From the Capital Beltway (I-495) in Oxon Hill, take Exit 2 or Exit 3 and the long exit ramp to get onto southbound MD 210 (Indian Head Highway). Proceed about 8.3 miles, and then turn right onto the exit ramp leading to Bryan Point Road. Follow the service road, and turn right onto Bryan Point Road. At the ALL VISITORS sign, turn right onto the gravel road and proceed 100 yards to the parking lot near the visitor center.

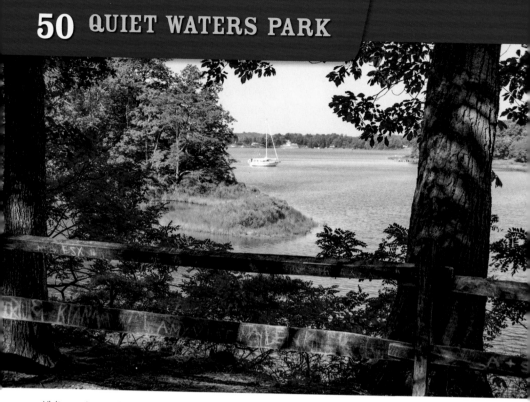

Visitors enjoy scenic views of the South River and Harness Creek.

WITH ITS PRIME LOCATION between the South River and Harness Creek near Annapolis, Quiet Waters Park offers 6 miles of trails that wind through forests and past scenic river overlooks.

DESCRIPTION

Quiet Waters was a farm that changed ownership many times prior to becoming a park. The property was a valuable plot of land divided into two primary estates in the 17th and 18th centuries: the Harness Estate and Hill's Delight. In 1987, the trustees of the Mary E. Parker Foundation sold the property to Anne Arundel County.

This hike is along a paved hiker-biker trail that traverses the full length of the 340-acre park, winding in and out of the woods. Begin your walk from the visitor center parking lot where you see an orange flag for biking and boat rentals. Follow the trail to the left. Turn left again after you pass the Dogwood picnic pavilion. As you pass the visitor center, take a look at the nicely manicured gardens. When you come to the trail crossing, turn right to stay on the trail; pass another intersection and continue straight. At the next crossing, turn right and reenter the woods. As you follow the trail, you will come to a scenic overlook of Harness Creek with a small picnic area.

LENGTH 4.9 miles

CONFIGURATION Loop

DIFFICULTY Easy

SCENERY Woodlands; panoramas of South River and Harness Creek

EXPOSURE Mostly shady; less so in winter

TRAFFIC Usually light; heavier on warm-weather weekends and holidays

TRAIL SURFACE Paved

HIKING TIME 2 hours

DRIVING DISTANCE 32 miles

SEASON Year-round

ACCESS Open 7 a.m.–sunset (closed on Tuesdays). There is an entrance fee of $6 per vehicle.

WHEELCHAIR TRAVERSABLE Yes

MAPS Anne Arundel County, tinyurl.com /quietwatersmap

FACILITIES Restrooms at multiple locations along the trail

CONTACT 410-222-1777

LOCATION Annapolis, Maryland

Continue along the trail until you see a sign to turn right to the South River Overlook. Be sure to take this short detour, as it has the best views in the park. There are two gazebos, many benches, and a large grassy area. From the overlook, walk back to the trail, and continue right. You will pass the fenced-in dog park with separate areas for large and small dogs. As you continue, you will see the park's concert stage on the left and some picnic tables. At this point, you will return to a crossing where you'll be doubling back to where you came from.

Turn right at the intersection, cross the maintenance road and continue straight. On your left you'll see the Blue Heron Center (an indoor event facility) and the Reading and Butterfly Gardens. Continue on the trail to enter the woods again. This part of the trail has exercise stations along the way. If you have the energy, try some pull-ups, parallel bars, or incline rings. When you come to the end of the fitness trail, cross the street and continue on the trail until you return to the parking lot.

NEARBY/RELATED ACTIVITIES

Kayaking and stand-up paddleboard tours and lessons are offered along Harness Creek and South River from mid-April through October. Reservations are required. Visit twistedcreekpaddlesports.com. Other recreational activities at the park include fishing, geocaching, and outdoor ice skating (in winter). Three art galleries are located in the visitor center: Willow Gallery, Garden Gallery, and Dogwood Gallery. They are open Monday, Wednesday, Thursday, and Friday 9 a.m.–4 p.m., and Saturday and Sunday, 10 a.m.–3 p.m. The park is located just 3 miles from downtown Annapolis, which offers a wide array of activities. Visit the waterfront for dining, shopping, boating excursions, and exploring historic sites.

Quiet Waters Park

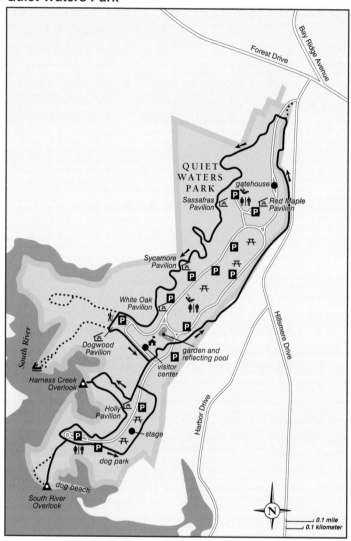

GPS TRAILHEAD COORDINATES N38° 56.289' W76° 30.303'

DIRECTIONS From I-495, take US 50 East, following the signs toward Annapolis. Take Exit 22 for MD 665 toward Aris T. Allen Boulevard/Riva Road; keep right to stay on Exit 22, following signs for MD 665 East/Riva Road. Follow MD 665 East and Forest Drive to Quiet Waters Park Road.

The park serves as a fine habitat for a variety of birds and woodland animals. Bird boxes are strategically set around the property to provide food and shelter for forest birds.

TUCKED AWAY IN A RURAL SECTION of Montgomery County, Rachel Carson Conservation Park is a hidden gem mostly used by local residents. The park is quiet and offers easy hiking trails with slight inclines and varying scenery.

DESCRIPTION

This small park honors Rachel Carson, the writer, environmental activist, and Montgomery County resident, by conserving 650 acres in the Brookeville area. It is also the proposed northern terminus for the Rachel Carson Greenway Trail, which, when completed, will span 25 miles, stretching from the historic Adelphi Mill in Prince George's County north to Patuxent River State Park. Some interpretive signs relating to the area's environmental, historical, and cultural heritage have been installed along the trail corridor. The trails are well marked, and county volunteers do a good job at maintaining this lightly used recreation area.

As the trail starts, you will be walking along Fox Meadow Loop, a wide grassy path along an open meadow with bird feeder boxes—a walk in these woods may offer a chance to see and hear forest birds such as the Kentucky warbler and ovenbird.

LENGTH 2.7 miles (with longer options, up to 6 miles)

CONFIGURATION Modified loop

DIFFICULTY Easy

SCENERY Rolling woodlands, streams, meadow

EXPOSURE Mostly shady and open (meadow only)

TRAFFIC Light

TRAIL SURFACE Dirt and grass (meadow only)

HIKING TIME 1.5 hours

DRIVING DISTANCE 39 miles

SEASON Year-round

ACCESS No restrictions

WHEELCHAIR TRAVERSABLE No

MAPS Montgomery Parks, montgomery parks.org

FACILITIES None

CONTACT Montgomery Parks, 301-495-2595

LOCATION Brookeville, Maryland

COMMENTS The trail is open to horses.

Turn right onto Rachel Carson Greenway Trail and enter the woods. When you come to the Fern Valley Trail, turn right to stay on Rachel Carson Greenway.

At the River Otter Trail, take a left and continue on Rachel Carson Greenway as you walk along the beautiful Hawlings River. You will see some evidence of flour mills that were once located along the stream valley. When you reach the intersection of Hidden Pond Trail, turn right to stay on Rachel Carson Greenway. The park is densely populated by numerous species of plants, including lush patches of skunk cabbage, a low-growing plant that occurs in wetlands of eastern North America. Turn left onto the Fern Valley Trail, after which the path starts to climb again.

At the next crossing make a right onto Chestnut Oak Trail, and keep right to stay on Chestnut Oak Trail. After a while, you'll come to the edge of the park, where there will be a fence and you can see the back of a farm with horses. Turn left to follow Chestnut Oak Trail. As you exit the woods, you'll reach the meadow. Turn left onto Fox Meadow Loop and continue back to the parking lot.

For a longer hike, check out some of the other trails. The Hidden Pond Trail leads to a small pond that teems with frogs during mating season. In summer, the eastern side of the Fox Meadow Loop grows beautiful swamp milkweed plants with pink blossoms that grow 4–5 feet tall.

NEARBY/RELATED ACTIVITIES

Located just a few miles away on Brookeville Road is Oakley Cabin (301-650-4373, montgomeryparks.org) a 19th-century African American historic site. Inhabited until 1976, the cabin is now operated by Montgomery Parks as a living history museum providing hands-on experiences. Also nearby, the Triadelphia Reservoir is a good spot for kayaking, fishing, and picnicking. For more information, visit wsscwater.com /watershedregs.

Rachel Carson Conservation Park

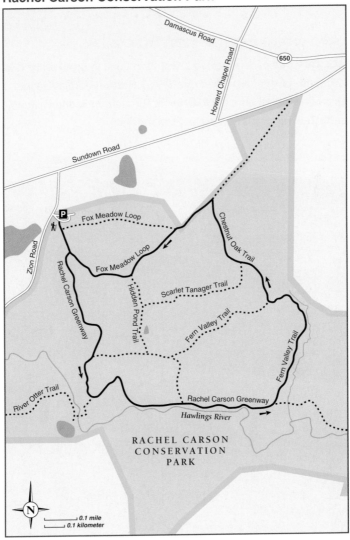

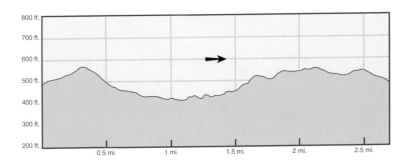

• •

GPS TRAILHEAD COORDINATES N39° 13.191' W77° 05.136'

DIRECTIONS The park is located 22201 Zion Road in Brookeville. It is east of I-270 and north of MD 200. From MD 97 North (Georgia Avenue), head north and take a left onto MD 650 North. Turn left on Sundown Road, then left onto Zion Road; the parking lot is on the left.

Rachel Carson Conservation Park offers more than 6 miles of natural-surface trails.

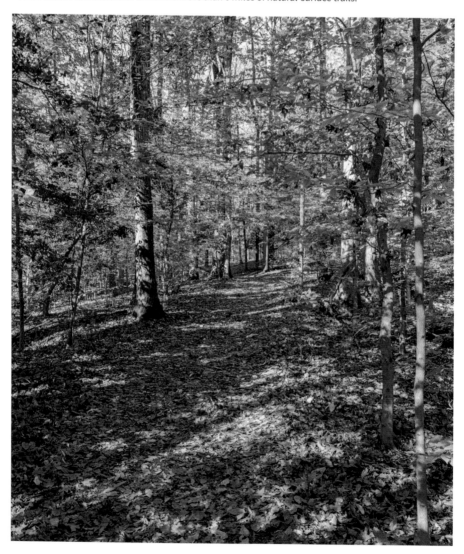

52 SUGARLOAF MOUNTAIN

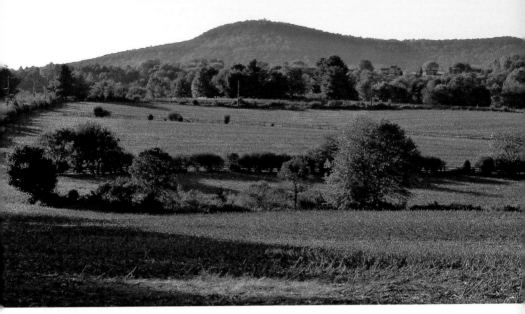

Sugarloaf Mountain, a rather small peak, is surrounded by farmland and is visible from many parts of Montgomery and Southern Frederick Counties.

WASHINGTON'S NEAREST MOUNTAIN is vista-rich Sugarloaf Mountain, located in southern Frederick County. You can hike up, around, and down it in half a day. You can also use the map to devise shorter or longer options.

DESCRIPTION

This 4.6-mile woodland hike is a clockwise loop featuring 814 feet of elevation change. The Mountain Loop Trail, designated with white blazes, starts from West View, the highest parking lot and picnic area. The trail remains level for a while as it traverses the backcountry, remaining predominantly in thick woods with rocky outcrops. The second half of the hike descends to the main entrance and then proceeds back up to the West View parking lot. The Potomac Appalachian Trail Club maintains these trails; most are blazed, color coded, and signposted but can still be confusing.

After arriving and picking up your trail map at the entrance, drive all the way up to the West View parking lot (you'll pass two other parking lots on the way up). Through the trees, you'll catch a glimpse of some gorgeous views of the surrounding farmland. Look for the Northern Peaks Trailhead at the edge of the parking lot,

LENGTH 3.8 miles (with longer and shorter options)

CONFIGURATION Loop

DIFFICULTY Moderate

SCENERY Upland woodlands, sweeping vistas, forest

EXPOSURE Mostly shady; less so in winter

TRAFFIC Usually light; crowded on warm-weather weekends, during fall foliage season, and on holidays, especially on and near the summit

TRAIL SURFACE Roughly half hard-packed dirt; rocky and rooty

HIKING TIME 2 hours

DRIVING DISTANCE 46 miles

SEASON Year-round

ACCESS Open daily, sunrise–sunset; road within park opens at 8 a.m. and closes 1 hour before sunset.

WHEELCHAIR TRAVERSABLE No

MAPS Stronghold Incorporated, tinyurl.com /sugarloafmtnmap

FACILITIES Water and phone at trailhead, with restroom nearby; restrooms at parking lots and entrance

CONTACT Stronghold Incorporated, 301-869-7846, sugarloafmd.com

LOCATION Dickerson, Maryland

marked with both blue and white blazes. Begin the trail by walking down the rocky, uneven steps. At the intersection of the two-in-one blue- and white-blazed trail, bear right, following the Mountain Loop Trail, marked with only white blazes. Keep following the white blazes, down man-made stone stairs and through trees and rocks covered in lichens. At a few points, the path has rocky outcrops with large boulders on either side, providing a fun place to climb around.

At the next intersection, you'll see that the white trail and blue trail diverge; you'll head right to follow the Mountain Loop Trail's white blazes. Shortly after that intersection, you'll encounter a trail marker; turn left to stay on the white-blazed trail. At this point, the trail continues on fairly level terrain, through pristine meadows of ferns underneath a conifer forest canopy.

After going down some stairs again, you'll see a signpost marking the northern split between the blue- and the white-blazed trails. Follow the white-blazed trail over some wooden planks. The path begins a descent on the edge of a ravine, with some views of the farmhouses in the distance. Follow the trail past the sign for the East View parking lot. Then cross the mountain road, remaining on the white trail.

The Mountain Loop Trail descends from 725 feet to 500 feet. You'll end up at a second road with a sign pointing right to stay on the white trail. The road jogs right for a few feet, and then you'll see you've reached the bottom of the mountain— the entrance to Sugarloaf Mountain near where you picked up the map. Follow the gravel road to the right toward the woods.

While you're at the foot of the mountain, you can stop at Strong Mansion. You'll see a portable toilet and a barn. Pass by the SMOKEY SAYS fire-prevention sign on the gravel road, and walk toward the trail marked by yellow and white blazes. Turn right

Sugarloaf Mountain

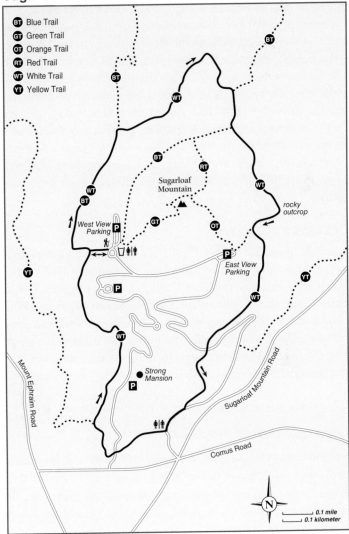

- **BT** Blue Trail
- **GT** Green Trail
- **OT** Orange Trail
- **RT** Red Trail
- **WT** White Trail
- **YT** Yellow Trail

Sugarloaf Mountain

rocky outcrop

West View Parking

East View Parking

Strong Mansion

Mount Ephraim Road

Sugarloaf Mountain Road

Comus Road

N

0.1 mile
0.1 kilometer

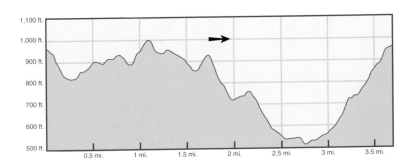

to follow the white trail and head back up the hill. This gravel and rocky trail is fairly steep as it climbs uphill 400 feet. Stay on this trail until you reach the intersection of the blue trail. Turn right and back up the steps to return to the West View parking lot. When you pass the Potomac Overlook parking sign, continue straight.

If you wish to reach the summit, it's a sharp 300-foot hike uphill on Thomas Trail from the West View parking area. Called Monadnock (geologically, Sugarloaf is a monadnock—an outlier of the Blue Ridge), the trail is marked with green blazes. It intersects the red and orange trails at the summit, a flat and massive rock slab covering about an acre. Head for the tree- and bush-rimmed edge in search of viewing spots. Also, climb the highest nearby rock; at 1,282 feet above sea level, you'll be some 800 feet above the surrounding farmlands. Retrace your steps back down to the parking lot.

NEARBY/RELATED ACTIVITIES

Stop at Sugarloaf Mountain Vineyard (301-605-0130, smvwinery.com), just a few miles from the entrance to Sugarloaf Mountain. The winery hosts tours and weekend events that are open to the public, including children. Continue north on Mount Ephraim Road to visit the Lilypons Water Gardens, which covers more than 300 seasonally colorful acres, sells aquatic plants and ornamental fish, and mounts public events. Still owned by the same family, the business was started as a goldfish farm in 1917 by an opera buff who later named it for renowned coloratura Lily Pons. For driving directions and the events schedule, call 800-999-5459 or visit lilypons.com.

• •

GPS TRAILHEAD COORDINATES N39° 15.699' W77° 23.828'

DIRECTIONS From the Capital Beltway (I-495), head northwest on I-270 (toward Frederick) 22 miles. Get off at Exit 22, turn right onto MD 109, and head west about 3 miles. Then turn right onto MD 95 (Comus Road) and proceed 2.5 miles to the small parking area at the base of the mountain, just outside the entrance gate.

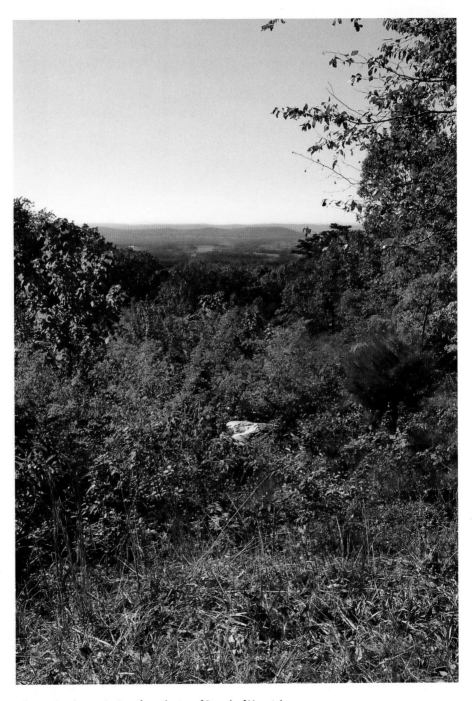

Hikers enjoy the scenic vistas from the top of Sugarloaf Mountain.

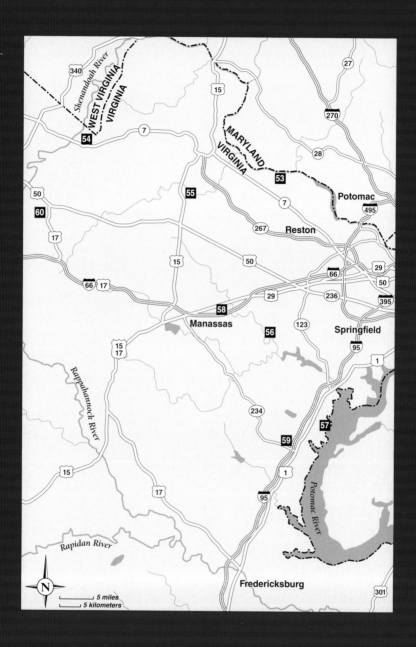

RURAL VIRGINIA
(Clarke, Fauquier, Loudoun, and Prince William Counties)

53 ALGONKIAN REGIONAL PARK

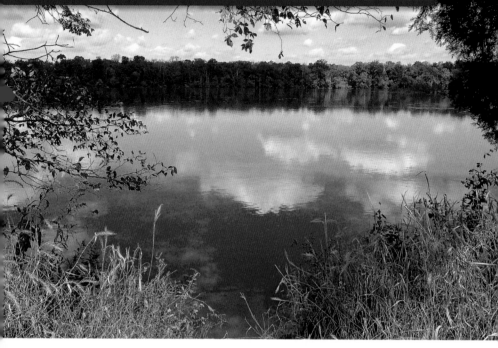

Stay overnight at Algonkian Park's Riverside Cabin to enjoy a weekend on the water.

LOUDOUN COUNTY'S REGIONAL PARK is chock-full of outdoor activities, including some protected nature preserves. Located on the Potomac River, the trail consists of shoreline strolls, forested paths, and wetland navigation.

DESCRIPTION

Algonkian Regional Park is one of Loudoun County's best-equipped outdoor recreation areas. Among the 838 acres of adventures, there is much to do year-round, from golf and tennis to boating and fishing, as well as semi-wheelchair-accessible hiking trails. The park rents cabins overlooking the Potomac River, so you could make a weekend of it.

Originally home to American Indian tribes, the property was a major route for settlers between Alexandria and the Shenandoah Valley. Part of the Algonkian landscape is a sanctuary for birds. The trails are concentrated in what is known as Lowes Island and the Potomac Heritage Trail (PHT). Incorporated into the Virginia Birding and Wildlife Trail, Algonkian is an excellent place to spot songbirds, dragonflies, and butterflies. A wildflower meadow contains the oldest bluebird-nest-box trail in the region. While exploring the wetlands, keep an eye out for herons, kingfishers, and

LENGTH 2.5 miles (with longer options)

CONFIGURATION Loop

DIFFICULTY Easy

SCENERY Wide river scenes, forest, streams, golf course, boat launch

EXPOSURE Shady; less so in winter

TRAFFIC Usually light; busier on warm-weather weekends

TRAIL SURFACE Mostly dirt or grass, with stretches of pavement and gravel; rocky in places

HIKING TIME 1–1.5 hours

DRIVING DISTANCE 33 miles

SEASON Year-round

ACCESS Open daily, sunrise–sunset

WHEELCHAIR TRAVERSABLE Partially

MAPS Available at visitor center

FACILITIES Restrooms, water, minigolf, picnic shelters, playground, riverfront cottages for rent, RV and boat storage, Volcano Waterpark, The Woodlands event facility, soccer fields

CONTACT NOVA Parks, 703-450-4655, novaparks.com

LOCATION Sterling, Virginia

COMMENTS Park is family friendly; cottages and campsites are available for overnights.

eagles; they thrive in this habitat. Besides a wide section of the Potomac River, the park contains vernal pools and a swamp that attracts a variety of amphibians.

Start your hike at the boat-launch parking lot; the trailhead is to the right. It begins on the PHT, which parallels the river. While walking along the riverside, stop at a few of the overlooks for wide-open views of tiny Sharpshin and Tenfoot Islands. Across the river, on the Maryland side, you can see the McKee-Beshers Wildlife Management Area and Seneca Creek State Park.

After a short walk, you end up next to the Algonkian Golf Course to your right. The trail is flat and easy here with some leafy coverage. Now and then you'll see the blue blazes designating the PHT. Soon the trail detours right and moves to the south side of the golf course. Veer off the PHT to stay on the north side of the course. Join the connector trail that intersects the Woodlands Trail. This is not a heavily forested area, and you can see the golf course as you hike on the connector.

Remaining on the Woodlands Trail, take the right fork into the Algonkian Sanctuary, a new-growth forest with wildflowers, oak trees, and wetlands. Soon you're deep enough to hear and see more birds, such as cardinals, blue jays, and woodpeckers.

Next the trail turns left, and you enter a grove of trees. This trail undulates like a roller coaster, and you'll pass some bluebird-nest boxes. Over by the stream called Sugarland Run, you might spot a hawk or heron languishing in the shady wetlands of the gully. The Sanctuary Trail is located on the other side of Sugarland Run, but unfortunately there's no way to access it from the Woodland Trail except from the PHT. So don't try to cross this stream; it's easy to fall in.

Algonkian Regional Park

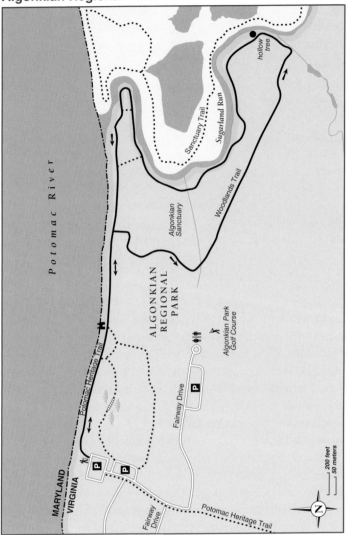

Continue down the Woodlands Trail, and you'll be walking to the left of Sugarland Run, a widening stream that eventually empties into the Potomac River. Again, keep following the blue blazes until the stream broadens and joins the river. Next there are a couple of quick turns made in succession. Turn right at the next intersection. Then take the right fork, and then a quick left fork to turn back toward the Potomac onto the Woodland Trail. Once back by the Potomac, retrace your steps to the parking lot.

NEARBY/RELATED ACTIVITIES

Consider playing minigolf or checking out Volcano Waterpark at Algonkian Regional Park in warm-weather months. Claude Moore Park is another nearby park with 357 acres; it has fields, an Olympic-size pool, and hiking trails. Check out Sugarland Park Shopping Center if you're looking for restaurants and shops. Frying Pan Park in Herndon offers families a visit to a 1920s to 1950s–style working farm with horses, pigs, tractor rides, and a merry-go-round. For more hiking, Algonkian is near Fraser Preserve (Hike 30, page 143) and Riverbend Park (Hike 37, page 174).

• •

GPS TRAILHEAD COORDINATES N39° 03.724' W77° 22.693'

DIRECTIONS From the Capital Beltway (I-495) take Exit 45A to merge onto VA 267 toward Dulles airport. Take Exit 16 to merge onto VA 7/Leesburg Pike north toward Leesburg (both VA 267 and VA 7 are toll roads). Take the ramp onto MD 6220/Algonkian Parkway. Turn right onto Cascades Parkway and drive 3.8 miles; it merges into Fairway Drive. Turn right into the park at 47001 Fairway Drive.

Adjacent to a golf course, Algonkian Sanctuary is a peaceful setting full of wildflowers, oak trees, and wetlands.

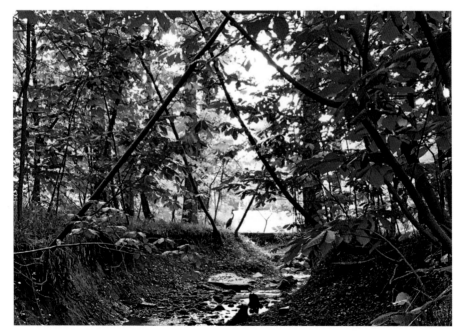

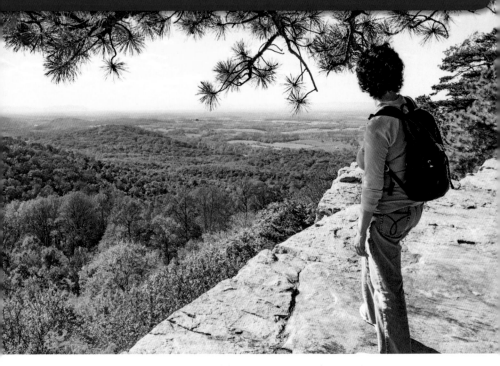

The Appalachian Trail provides spectacular hiking opportunities with scenic vistas.

ON THIS BEAUTIFUL SEGMENT of the Appalachian Trail, hikers wind up and down through a variety of terrain, visiting two states (Virginia and West Virginia) and crossing a rocky ridge to a scenic vista.

DESCRIPTION

The Georgia-to-Maine Appalachian Trail (AT) was conceived in the 1920s by a forester, planner, and visionary named Benton MacKaye. A primitive version was in place by 1937, but it took decades to refine the route, secure public ownership, and arrange permanent maintenance. Now officially called the Appalachian National Scenic Trail and under National Park Service administration, the 2,168-mile trail is managed by the Appalachian Trail Conservancy (ATC) and maintained by local organizations and their volunteers. The Potomac Appalachian Trail Club (PATC), for example, takes care of the AT and its side trails throughout the mid-Atlantic states.

Raven Rocks is a 5.2-mile hike in what is referred to as "the roller-coaster section" of the AT, an up-and-down, rocky path that offers challenging hiking and leads to panoramic views of the Shenandoah Valley and Blue Ridge Mountains. The hike begins at a trailhead off of Pine Grove Road (at the intersection of VA 7) in Bluemont, Virginia. There is no sign designating the trail name, but the trailhead is

LENGTH 5.2 miles (with longer options)

CONFIGURATION Out-and-back

DIFFICULTY Moderately challenging

SCENERY Mountain woodlands; panoramic vista at the summit

EXPOSURE Mostly shady; less so in winter

TRAFFIC Moderate; heavier on warm-weather weekends and holidays

TRAIL SURFACE Mostly dirt and rocks, with rooty patches

HIKING TIME 4 hours

DRIVING DISTANCE 60 miles

SEASON Year-round, best in spring and fall on a clear day so you can appreciate the views

ACCESS No restrictions

WHEELCHAIR TRAVERSABLE No

MAPS Potomac Appalachian Trail Club (PATC) Map 7

FACILITIES None

CONTACT Appalachian Trail Conservancy, 717-258-5771, appalachiantrail.org

LOCATION Bluemont, Virginia

COMMENTS Be careful, as this is a rocky ramble that requires agility. Avoid hiking after rainy weather, when the trail is slippery and dangerous. Be sure to give yourself enough time to return before dark. This hike is not appropriate for young children.

obvious. When you see the white blazes on the left, you will know you are at the right place. You can also begin the hike from Bears Den, the historic lodge nearby, adding 0.8 mile each way to the hike. See more about Bears Den at the end of this profile.

The steep, rocky trail (with more than 1,500 feet of elevation change) zigzags between Virginia and West Virginia and is shaded by oaks, hickories, beeches, and maples. This section is famous for its hilly terrain and offers some of the most challenging hiking in the area. The trail begins with a slow incline and then goes downhill for most of the first mile. Remember to save your energy, as this means you will be climbing uphill at the end of the hike. The trail is well marked with white blazes and is easy to follow. It makes several steep switchback descents and involves some scrambling over large boulders and mossy, rocky terrain. Be sure to wear sturdy footwear, and carry a walking stick if you like the support and stability.

As you climb the final ascent to the summit, you'll pass a sign marking the Virginia–West Virginia border. Raven Rocks is a spur of the Blue Ridge Mountain in Jefferson County, West Virginia. The peak is located just north of Clarke County, Virginia, and west of its border with Loudoun County, Virginia. When you reach the summit, enjoy 180-degree views of the rolling hills and farms of the Shenandoah Valley. Rest awhile and eat your lunch before retracing your steps back to the parking lot.

NEARBY/RELATED ACTIVITIES

The nearby Bears Den, (540-554-8708, bearsdencenter.org) is a popular stopover for AT thru-hikers. There are a number of easy hikes as well as a scenic overlook that is a great place to watch the sunset. Amenities include a bathroom, lodge, and camping

Appalachian Trail: Raven Rocks

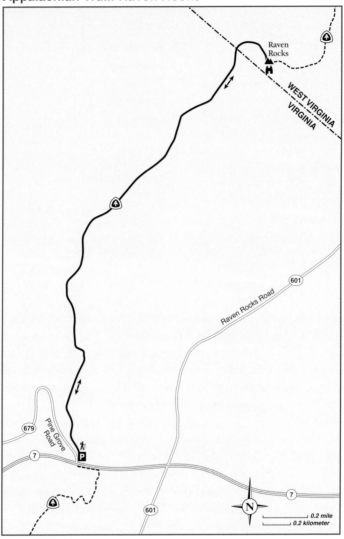

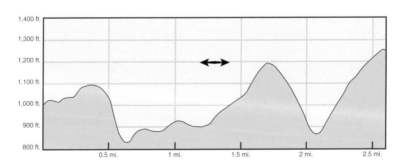

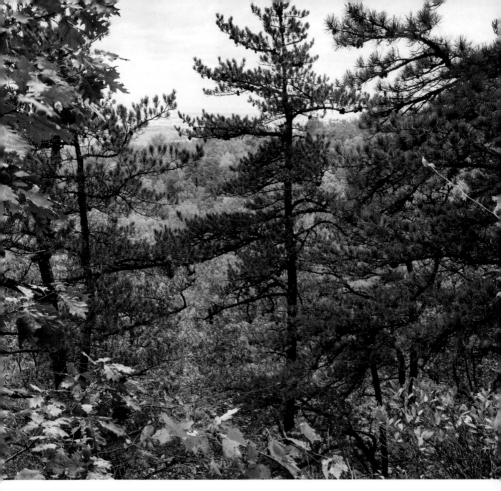

The Ravens Rock Trail is shaded by oak, hickory, beech, and maple trees.

and picnic areas. There is a $3 honor system–based entrance fee. Stop at Horse Shoe Curve (540-554-8291) or Pine Grove Restaurant (540-554-8126, pinegrove restaurant.webstarts.com) for a bite after your hike. Twin Oaks Tavern Winery (540-554-4547, twinoakstavernwinery.com) is just across VA 7 up Raven Rocks Road, less than 5 minutes away, and Veramar Vineyard is east on VA 7, about 10 minutes away.

• •

GPS TRAILHEAD COORDINATES N39° 06.992' W77° 51.141'

DIRECTIONS From the Capital Beltway (I-495), follow VA 267 West to US 15 South/VA 7 West/Leesburg Bypass. Follow VA 7 west 19 miles to VA 679/Pine Grove Road. The parking lot and trailhead are on the right just off of VA 7. The parking lot has limited space, and street parking is not permitted in front of the trailhead. Alternatively, park about 0.2 mile farther down Pine Grove Road, past the NO PARKING signs, or in the overflow lot across VA 7, if necessary.

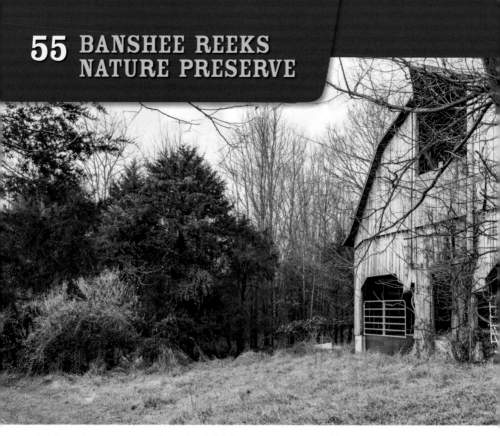

This lesser-known preserve offers a delightful place to enjoy nature and farmland scenery.

WITH MORE THAN A DOZEN HIKING TRAILS totaling 20 miles among rolling hills and frontage along Goose Creek, Banshee Reeks is Loudoun County's only nature preserve. Most of the trails are short and can be combined to create a loop.

DESCRIPTION

Why does this beautiful place have such a funny name? The word *banshee* is a Gaelic term for a female spirit and the word *reeks* is a Gaelic term for hills and dales. Legend has it that in the early part of the 19th century, the owner of the farm, who was of Irish or Scottish descent, heard strange cries and sounds in the woods and referred to them as "banshees in the reeks."

The 775-acre nature preserve is run by volunteers and owned by the Loudoun County Department of Parks, Recreation & Community Services. It is located in the Piedmont region of Virginia, which stretches from the falls of the Potomac, Rappahannock, and James Rivers to the Blue Ridge Mountains. While many of its neighboring areas are facing urban sprawl, the lush landscape here retains its rural personality. The villages, farms, vineyards, and churchyards set on rolling hills and tucked into valleys are reminiscent of rural England.

LENGTH 3.6 miles (with shorter and longer options)

CONFIGURATION Loop

DIFFICULTY Easy

SCENERY Hardwood forests, wetlands, fields, ponds, streams

EXPOSURE Shady; less so in winter

TRAFFIC Mostly very light–light; heavier on warm-weather weekends and holidays

TRAIL SURFACE Grass and dirt

HIKING TIME 2 hours

DRIVING DISTANCE 42 miles

SEASON Year-round, but best in spring and fall

ACCESS Open weekends only, 8 a.m.–4 p.m. Other times by appointment. The visitor center is open on the third weekend of each month.

WHEELCHAIR TRAVERSABLE No

MAPS Sketch maps in a box in front of visitor center; tinyurl.com/bansheemap

FACILITIES Portable toilet at visitor center

LOCATION Leesburg, Virginia

CONTACT Friends of Banshee Reeks, 703-669-0316, bansheereeksnp.org; Loudoun County Department of Parks, Recreation & Community Services, 703-777-0343, loudoun.gov/prcs

COMMENTS Take only pictures and leave only footprints. The preserve allows leashed dogs, but horses and bikes are not permitted.

Banshee Reeks protects native plants and animals in many different habitats, including mixed hardwood forests of oak and hickory, fields, ponds, streams, hedgerows, meadows, and wetlands. Wildlife includes beavers, deer, foxes, numerous species of birds, amphibians, reptiles, and insects.

The manor house contains the staff offices and the visitor center, which serves as a nature center. In 2015, the display room was refurbished with museum-quality specimens of local flora and fauna. Families can enjoy the books, games, and puzzles in the reception area. There is also a honeybee display with a visible hive and a collection of taxidermy and animal bones. An 1830s log cabin and bank barn are also located on the property. Goose Creek flows for more than 2 miles along the southern border of the property. Public programs and nature walks are offered year-round by various wildlife organizations, schools, and facility staff. A primitive camping area is available for Boy Scouts and Girl Scouts, by special permit only.

This 3.6-mile hike is easy, with a variety of scenery. You can create a shorter or a longer hike depending on your interest and ability. From the visitor center, start by turning left onto the gravel road. Continue past the first trail sign, and walk toward the grain silos. Turn left onto the Greenway Trail, a grass path that winds through the center of the preserve past several merging trails. Keep straight, following the signs for the Greenway Trail, until you reach a barn with a road to the left of it. Turn right onto the Bankbarn Trail and walk just over 100 feet; then turn left onto the Wetlands Trail. This trail runs along the southeastern edge of the park and leads to Goose Creek.

As you walk along the creek, when you get to an intersection, continue straight past Bankbarn Trail and then again as the trail merges onto Eastern Watercress Trail. When the trail ends, turn left onto Western Watercress Trail. Cross the stream by

Banshee Reeks Nature Preserve

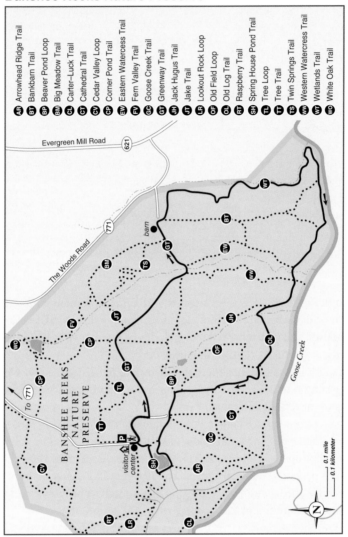

hopping over a few rocks, and continue up a hill. Then turn left onto Jack Hugus Trail. Turn left again to take the Old Log Trail, crossing the stream again, then proceeding up a slightly steeper hill.

As you cross a few more intersections, continue straight as the trail merges into Old Field Loop. After another intersection with Old Log Trail, turn right at an unmarked trail, and continue to the intersection with Beaver Pond Loop; turn left. Continue walking past the grain silos on your right. Keep straight behind the barn as you see views of the mountains and the manor house (visitor center).

As you pass the maintenance barn, the trail becomes Goose Creek Trail, and then at the bottom of the hill it becomes Spring House Trail. At the giant white oak, turn left to visit Spring House Pond. Follow the trail around to the left, circling the pond. Be sure to enjoy the views, as this is one of the most scenic spots in the park. At the far end of the pond, continue straight to the end of the fence, and then make a right back onto Spring House Trail. Follow the trail to the next intersection, and make a left on the unmarked trail to head back to the visitor center and parking lot.

NEARBY/RELATED ACTIVITIES

The park is about 6 miles south of the town of Leesburg. After your hike, explore the historic district and enjoy shopping or dining, or visit one of the many wineries in Loudoun County. Kids will enjoy a stop at Leesburg Animal Park (703-433-0002, leesburganimalpark.com), a petting zoo where you can get up close to zebras, lemurs, camels, and other exotic animals. Or visit Morven Park (703-777-2414, morvenpark.org), a 1,000-acre historic estate and equestrian park with English gardens and the Winmill Carriage Museum.

• •

GPS TRAILHEAD COORDINATES N39° 01.693' W77° 35.994'

DIRECTIONS From the Capital Beltway (I-495), take the Dulles Access Road (VA 267) west to Exit 3, VA 653/Shreve Mill Road. Follow VA 653 west 0.9 mile. Turn left on Evergreen Mills Road, and follow it 2.5 miles. Turn right on VA 771/The Woods Road. The entrance to Banshee Reeks is on the right.

The manor house at Banshee Reeks sits atop a hill and has beautiful views of the surrounding farmland.

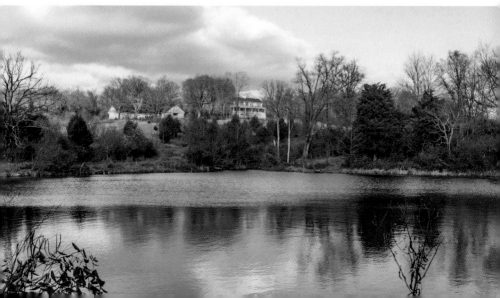

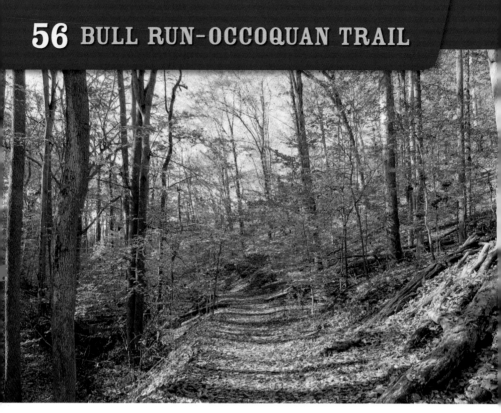

The Bull Run–Occoquan Trail is especially beautiful in fall when the leaves change color.

THE 18-MILE TRAIL WINDS THROUGH four adjoining parks in southwestern Fairfax County, Virginia, providing a picturesque hike. The 5-mile stretch described here, starting at Hemlock Overlook Regional Park, is one of the prettiest sections as it runs close to the Occoquan Reservoir.

DESCRIPTION

For a very scenic hike within an hour's drive of Washington, D.C., this one-way, 18-mile trek on the Bull Run–Occoquan Trail offers as rigorous a hike as anyone may want. Located about 25 miles southwest of the city, the trail is the only one in the area on which you can hike in roughly the same direction for 18 miles in a rural setting. That will take you from Bull Run Regional Park to Fountainhead Regional Park. For a shorter hike, you can do an out-and-back hike from any of the four parks along the way. The trail follows the valley carrying Bull Run and the Occoquan River to the Potomac River. It winds through wooded hills and floodplains and is marked by a rich assortment of flora and fauna, including large stands of hemlocks and spring-time bluebells. Before setting out, check trail conditions by calling 703-352-5900. Plan to follow the blue-blazed trail and its double-sided mileposts giving distances from each end.

LENGTH 5 miles (with longer and shorter options)

CONFIGURATION Out-and-back

DIFFICULTY Moderate

SCENERY Wooded hills, stream valleys, floodplains

EXPOSURE Shady; less so in winter

TRAFFIC Mostly very light–light; heavier on warm-weather weekends and holidays

TRAIL SURFACE Mostly dirt; rocks, gravel

HIKING TIME 2.5 hours

DRIVING DISTANCE 32 miles

SEASON Year-round

ACCESS Open daily, sunrise–sunset

WHEELCHAIR TRAVERSABLE No

MAPS Northern Virginia Regional Park Authority, novaparks.com

FACILITIES None

CONTACT Northern Virginia Regional Park Authority, 703-352-5900, novaparks.com

LOCATION Clifton, Virginia

COMMENTS As this is a very long trail, you can access it from multiple destinations and take a short or an extensive hike. Trailheads and parking lots are located at Bull Run Regional Park, Hemlock Overlook Regional Park, Bull Run Marina, and Fountainhead Regional Park.

To get started from Hemlock Overlook Regional Park, park at the lot on Yates Ford Road. The parking area is directly across from the Paradise Springs Winery. The park is also home to an outdoor education center operated by Adventure Links, which provides ropes courses, team-building programs, and adventure camps for youth. Pass the wooden posts and follow the yellow-blazed trail about a mile until you reach the reservoir. Turn left to head east. After passing through a rocky section, the trail follows the meandering stream across the floodplain. It then swings left and uphill into the woods, and the terrain becomes easier. Follow the blue blazes as the trail undulates for miles on dirt paths. Continue as far as you would like, and then follow the trail back to your starting point. Note: As you hike east, you may hear gunfire, as sound tends to travel down the valley from the Bull Run Shooting Range in Centreville, several miles away. To avoid the disturbance, check the website for hours, novaparks.com/parks/bull-run-shooting-center.

NEARBY/RELATED ACTIVITIES

After your hike, enjoy a glass of wine at the Paradise Springs Winery. It is open daily, 11 a.m.–7 p.m. (11 a.m.–9 p.m. on Friday). The property features an 18th-century log cabin, which was renovated in 1955 by a protégé of Frank Lloyd Wright.

Visit Bull Run Regional Park in April to see the Virginia bluebells in bloom. Take your own walk and time, or go on the annual, ranger-led Bluebell Walk. Call the park for details, 703-631-0550.

Visit the Manassas Industrial School/Jennie Dean Memorial in nearby Manassas. The memorial commemorates northern Virginia's first African American school and its remarkable founder, born a slave, who opened it as a private boarding school in

Bull Run–Occoquan Trail

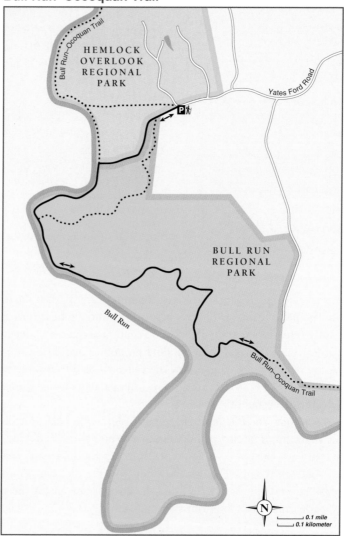

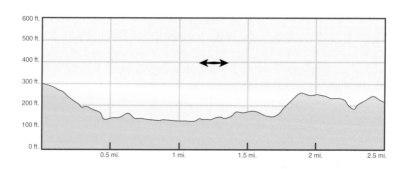

1894. For information and directions, contact the Manassas Museum, 703-368-1873, manassasmuseum.org.

In May and June, experience the vivid colors and fragrances of 200 old-rose varieties at the garden at Ben Lomond Historic Site in Manassas to. For information and directions, call 703-368-8784 or visit tinyurl.com/benlomondhistoricsite.

• •

GPS TRAILHEAD COORDINATES N38° 45.977' W77° 24.420'

DIRECTIONS From the Capital Beltway (I-495), take I-66 West to Exit 55 for Fairfax County Parkway South toward Springfield. After about 2 miles take the Braddock Road exit. Turn right onto Braddock Road and go about 2 miles. Turn left onto Clifton Road and drive about 3.5 miles. Bear right as you come into the town of Clifton. Go over the railroad tracks, through the town, and straight through the stop sign. Turn right onto Yates Ford Road. The parking lot will be on your right at the end of the road after about 1.5 miles.

The Occoquan River provides endless miles of beautiful scenery.

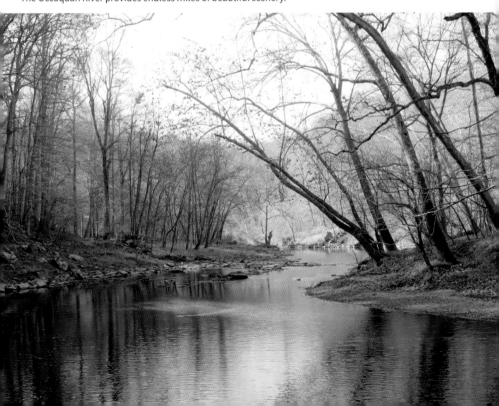

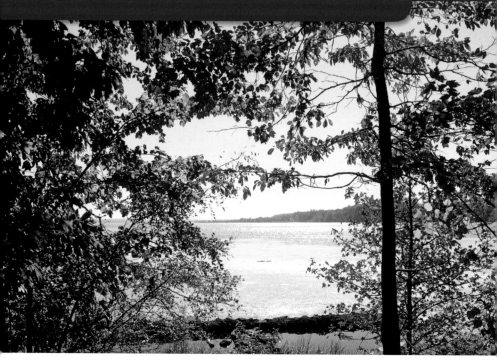

Leesylvania State Park is named for owner Harry Lighthorse Lee, who was a Revolutionary War hero. He was the father of Confederate general Robert E. Lee.

IN SOUTHEASTERN PRINCE WILLIAM COUNTY, Leesylvania State Park is a place where hikers can commune with nature, admire the Potomac River, and visit sites associated with Virginia's Lee family.

DESCRIPTION

Leesylvania State Park lies on a peninsula on the Potomac River in the Cherry Hill area, about 25 miles southwest of Washington. Its landscape features wooded uplands, wetlands, coastal bluffs, a sandy beach, and hiking trails. Trees and wildflowers flourish there, as do deer, beavers, and other four-footed creatures. Faunawatchers, though, mostly prize the eagles, ospreys, ducks, cormorants, and herons.

The park's history begins in the 1750s, when Henry Lee II developed a plantation called Leesylvania. One of the children born and reared there was Henry Lee III, the Light-Horse Harry of American Revolution fame. The property stayed in the family's hands until 1825. But the Lee link was revived during the Civil War, when General Robert E. Lee installed a gun battery here to block Union soldiers from accessing Washington, D.C. For a century thereafter, the area was used by tobacco farmers, loggers, fishermen, traders, squatters, hunters, and gambling-ship operators. In the late 1970s, philanthropist and playwright Daniel Ludwig acquired much

LENGTH 3.1 miles (with longer options)

CONFIGURATION Modified out-and-back

DIFFICULTY Easy–moderate

SCENERY Wooded uplands, wetlands, river and beach views

EXPOSURE Shady; less so in winter

TRAFFIC On riverfront, mostly heavy on warm-weather weekends and holidays; much lighter on weekdays and in winter

TRAIL SURFACE Mostly dirt; some board-walk, pavement, gravel, pebbles, sand

HIKING TIME 1.5 hours

DRIVING DISTANCE 30 miles

SEASON Year-round; best late fall–early spring

ACCESS Open daily, sunrise–sunset; entrance fee

WHEELCHAIR TRAVERSABLE Partially

MAPS Virginia Department of Conservation & Recreation, tinyurl.com/leesylvaniaspmap

FACILITIES Restrooms, water at park office (near trailhead); restrooms, water, phone, warm-season food store on riverfront; water at Freestone Point

CONTACT 703-730-8205, dcr.virginia.gov

LOCATION Woodbridge, Virginia

COMMENTS In addition to hearing the vroom-vroom of summer boats, you'll hear the whistle from the train.

of the area and donated it to the State of Virginia with support from the Society of Lees of Virginia group. The park was opened in 1992.

The 542-acre park is a popular warm-season destination for boaters and beach-goers. The riverfront gets crowded, and the boat engines roar. The shoreline has begun eroding, so the State of Virginia is building jetties parallel to the shoreline and covering them with aquatic plants. As the roots grow, they'll hold the sand in place, protecting the shoreline from additional erosion.

Leesylvania Park is one of the top destinations in Virginia for eagle-spotting. The park is at its colorful best in the spring and fall, and some winter days can be starkly beautiful. This 3.5-mile hike, with only about 500 feet of elevation change, includes two short trails and other paths. The trails are named and signposted, and most inter-sections are color coded and blazed, so it's easy to find your way. Take some time to listen and watch for wildlife on the many benches perched along the trails.

Get started at the Bushey Point trailhead by parking in the boater's lot (the first row is for cars, and the rest of the spaces are for trailers). At the kiosk, read about the 20-station fitness trail with exercises posted along the first leg of your journey. If you're feeling energetic, you might want to attempt a few calisthenics.

The hike travels west on a gently rising, hard-packed, sandy trail passing Fit-Trail signboards. As it proceeds through the woods, you'll see the Potomac River to your left. Take note of the duck blind and sign describing how this plantation produced tobacco in the 1700s. Fifty-five enslaved people lived and worked on this farm. There's a bench here, with views of the railroad bridge crossing the Potomac.

Follow the green blazes as the Bushey Point Trail enters the wetlands; there is a boardwalk built over them. Look for wildlife, including birds, frogs, and turtles. At

Leesylvania State Park

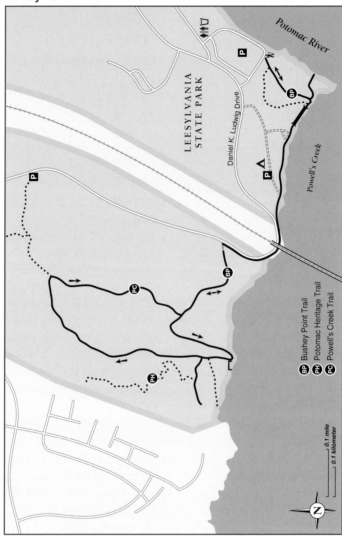

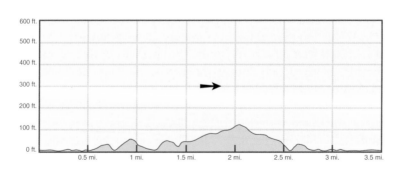

the next clearing, you'll see a boathouse with some canoes you can rent and a dock to put in. Walk underneath the railroad bridge, and then along Ludwig Drive a few feet until Bushey Point Trail reenters the forest. Take the trail left down some stairs, following the green blazes until you come to the Powell's Creek Trail. This trail forms a 1.28-mile loop through the woods. Take the trail left toward the Potomac Heritage Trail (PHT), which is marked with white blazes.

You'll go down some steep stairs, then curve left at the bottom, where you'll cross a gully on a small bridge. Stay with the trail as it takes you up a moderately steep hill to another set of stairs. At the top, just over a mile into the hike, you'll find a bench and trail junction. Continue straight on the green-blazed Bushey Point Trail (to the left is the Powell's Creek Trail's return loop).

At this point, you're approaching the peninsula created by the Potomac River and Powell's Creek. The scenic marshland, the tidal pools, and a beaver dam can be seen from the top of Cockpit Point from a bench with 180-degree views of the peninsula. Take a moment to survey your surroundings. These waters are known for their abundant freshwater fish, including largemouth bass.

At the next intersection you'll see a trail heading left toward the PHT and right to stay on Powell's Creek Trail. Take a quick detour left to explore the PHT, and then return to the intersection and rejoin Powell's Creek Trail as it heads deeper into the woods, away from the shoreline.

Follow the blue blazes and notice the many signs created by local high school students describing the wildlife typically found in the park. This trail is mostly flat and easy to navigate. Keep an eye out for woodpeckers and the five-lined skink, a lizard that lives in these woods.

Soon you'll come to white and blue blazes at the intersection of Powell's Creek Trail. Here you'll retrace your steps back to the parking lot. As you walk along the beach, do not be tempted to swim, as the water here is unsafe. When you pass under the Powell's Creek Bridge, you may see a train crossing. The original bridge, constructed of heavy timber, was 1,100 feet and built in 1872 with the aid of the Pennsylvania Railroad. The current bridge was rebuilt out of concrete to allow for longer, faster trains.

NEARBY/RELATED ACTIVITIES

Visit the Leesylvania Visitor Center (summer only) to see its absorbing history and science exhibits. Attend the annual Leesylvania Natural Heritage Day, held in May (contact the park for details). Visit the impressive National Museum of the Marine Corps in Triangle. The modern museum offers interpretive and living-history experiences with hands-on activities kids love. Consider taking a boat ride with Rivershore Charters, or go shopping at the popular Potomac Mills Outlet Mall. The Rippon Lodge Historic Site and Occoquan Bay National Wildlife Refuge are also worth a visit.

• •

GPS TRAILHEAD COORDINATES N38° 35.131' W77° 15.420'

DIRECTIONS From the Capital Beltway (I-495) in Springfield, Virginia, take Exit 57A onto I-95 heading southwest toward Richmond. If you start from Washington, head southwest on I-395 to automatically be on I-95 when you cross the Beltway. After going about 13 miles on I-95, watch for the Leesylvania State Park sign, and take Exit 156 to go west on VA 784 (Dale Boulevard). Go 0.7 mile, turn right onto Neabsco Mills Road, and proceed 1.1 miles. Turn right onto US 1 and get in the left lane; after 0.3 mile, turn left onto Neabsco Road. Go east 1.5 miles and turn right onto the park's access road; go 0.6 mile to the contact station and then to the gravel parking lot on the right—the trailhead. If it's full, go on to the next lot.

Leesylvania State Park trails offer picturesque overlooks of the Potomac River and are a haven for wildlife.

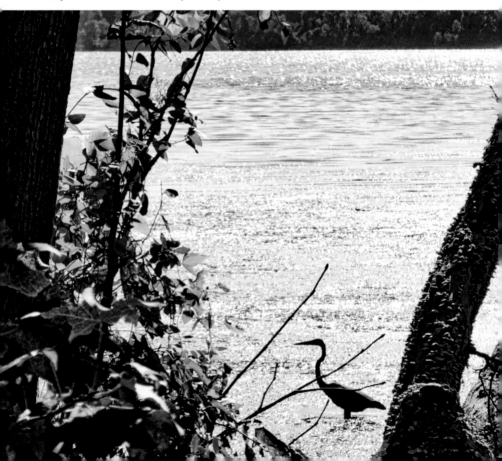

58 MANASSAS NATIONAL BATTLEFIELD PARK

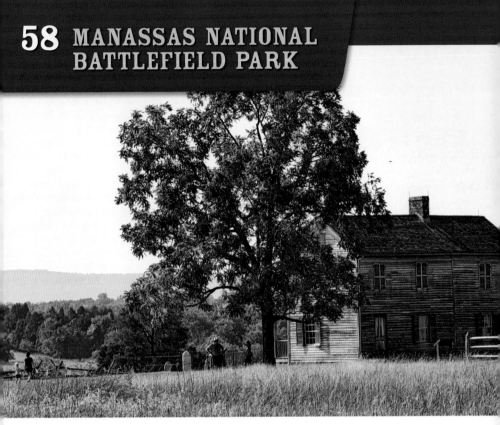

Manassas National Battlefield is day trip back in history. The collection of trails conjures images of the hardships troops faced during the two Civil War battles fought here.

A FEW MILES FROM HISTORIC MANASSAS, the National Park Service operates a multifaceted Civil War Battlefield experience with several short and long trail options for touring the sites. Stop at Henry Hill Visitor Center to learn about the significance of battles here before heading out on the trail.

DESCRIPTION

The Manassas battlefields are very accessible and lively, with a steady stream of visitors and recreation seekers. This lovingly cared-for national park encompasses 5,300 acres enshrining two significant Civil War battles. The first Manassas battle, also known as the First Battle of Bull Run, took place in July 1861. The soldiers of a divided nation had little experience with war at this point and enthusiastically gathered on the hills of Bull Run. During this violent, destructive one-day battle, the Union Army was defeated, with 4,878 casualties representing both sides. The second Manassas battle took place in August 1862—a rematch of sorts involving a seasoned army of soldiers with realistic expectations about the potential carnage that lay ahead. Three days later, the combined armies incurred 24,056 casualties. Once again,

LENGTH 5.4 miles (with shorter options)

CONFIGURATION Loop

DIFFICULTY Moderate

SCENERY Hilly woodlands, battlefield, river, wetlands, stone bridge, interpretive signs, ruins

EXPOSURE Exposed; some shady parts

TRAFFIC Moderate; busy on weekends and holidays

TRAIL SURFACE Gravel, dirt, grass, with stretches of boardwalk; rocky in places

HIKING TIME 3 hours

DRIVING DISTANCE 55 miles

SEASON Year-round, except Thanksgiving and Christmas Day

ACCESS Open daily, sunrise–sunset

WHEELCHAIR TRAVERSABLE On the boardwalk

MAPS National Park Service, tinyurl.com /manassasnbpmap

FACILITIES Restrooms, movie, water fountain, gift shop, museum, ranger information station, visitor center, additional satellite parking around battlefield

CONTACT National Park Service, 703-361-1339, nps.gov/mana

LOCATION Manassas, Virginia

COMMENTS Find a wide array of historic sites along the trails; expect intense sun exposure; dogs must be leashed; bicycles are prohibited; no climbing on structures; can be buggy in the summer.

the Confederate Army, led by Confederate generals Robert E. Lee and Stonewall Jackson, were victorious.

There are monuments and interpretive signs positioned strategically throughout the battlefield. Many of the buildings standing on this land were used as hospitals for the wounded. The preservation efforts have kept the scenery looking quite similar to how people saw it during those bloody years of war.

Before starting out, stop at the Henry Hill Visitor Center to pick up a trail map and, if you have time, watch the 45-minute video portraying the battles. There are multiple trail options ranging from 1 to 6 miles. Look for the sign to the First Manassas Battle trailhead on the edge of the parking lot, and start heading across the lawn. You'll see the Henry House to your left and a line of artillery directly in front of you.

You'll also see a statue of Stonewall Jackson on his horse. The line of artillery represents "Jackson's Line" from Confederate general Barnard Bee's famous quote. Bee shouted to his men about the newly arrived brigade led by General Jackson: "There stands Jackson like a stonewall! Rally behind the Virginians!"

After crossing the grassy meadow, you'll see another sign for the First Manassas Battle Trail pointing straight into the trees. The Henry Hill Loop Trail intersects here. After you pass that first sign, the trail becomes gravel. Note that much of this hike is open to direct sun, so you may want to avoid coming here in the heat of summer. The open fields remind hikers that both battles were fought in the region's hottest months, which must have added greatly to the suffering.

Manassas National Battlefield Park

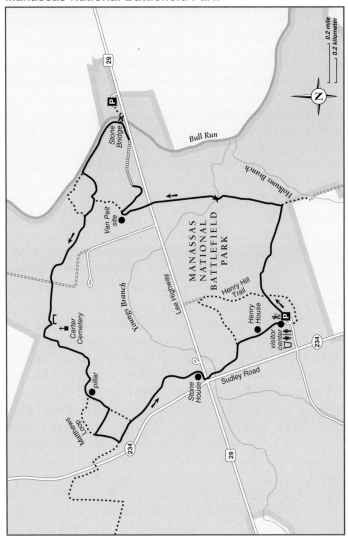

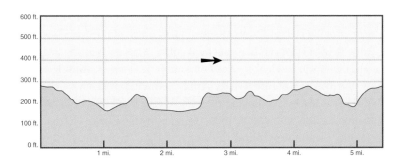

After the second trail marker you will start walking through thick woods with blue blazes on the trees. The forest consists of mostly young-growth trees; the land was a plantation and farmland before the battle occurred. Next you'll cross two small footbridges and then come to a sign indicating Stone Bridge to the left and Portici to the right. Turn left, following the blue blazes as the trail continues into the woods on a gravel path. On your left, you'll see a mulched path called the Bridle Trail. It's meant for horses, but a lot of runners use it.

The next intersection is confusing. Follow the signs for the First Manassas Battle Trail, making a left and then a quick jog to the right on the Van Pelt property. Right after, you'll cross Youngs Branch stream; you'll be walking north toward US 29 and will see the traditional wooden fences marking the Manassas Battlefield property. In this forest, you may see birds and deer.

As you approach US 29, the trail veers left at the fork, and you'll need to cross US 29 very carefully to rejoin the trail on the other side of the road. At the top of hill, the trail opens up to a panoramic view of the woods and fields spread across this property. You'll see a sign describing the Van Pelt house, where 70-year-old New Jersey native Abraham Van Pelt (nicknamed Yankee Van Pelt), his wife, his mother, and his daughter Elizabeth were forced to host Confederate Colonel Nathan G. Evans, who was deployed here during the first Manassas battle to guard the Stone Bridge. During the second battle, the Union soldiers commandeered the house, transforming it into a hospital. Throughout the conflict, the Van Pelts remained in their home. They were staunch Unionists, differing greatly in their adopted home from most of their neighbors on the Confederate side.

If at the fork you go straight, you'll cut off some hiking time. Otherwise head right to see the Stone Bridge following the blue blazes through a wheat field and into the woods. This bridge is where the opening shots were fired during the First Battle of Manassas. The Federals sent artillery shells into the Confederate camp at first light on July 21, 1861.

At the bottom of the hill you'll come to a long boardwalk built over wetlands where you'll probably see lots of joggers and dog walkers because there's a parking lot nearby. After the boardwalk you'll head toward Stone Bridge, walking beside US 29. As you walk along, be mindful of the occasional horse droppings on the trail.

Turn left just before Stone Bridge to walk on the west side of Bull Run. Walking beside the slow-moving river, follow the blue blazes up a couple dozen stairs to the end of the Stone Bridge Loop Trail. Next you'll come to a sign pointing out the ruins of Pittsylvania plantation, owned by Landon Carter Jr. There's nothing left of the mansion now, but you can see the Carter family cemetery. Otherwise continue on the trail marked NO HORSES, following the blue blazes into the woods again. Next you'll pass an intersection with a stone pillar designating the Eighth Georgia Infantry at Matthews Loop. Continue to follow the blue trail signs, crossing over a small platform to a clearing. Head toward the fences by walking up Matthews Hill.

Make a left when you see the Rhode Island Infantry sign to cut across Buck Hill field on a grassy trail. Far in the distance, you can see the visitor center. Pass through a line of artillery as you approach MD 234. At the last cannon, turn left and walk toward the visitor center. The trail is no longer marked, so just follow the trodden path.

Make your way down the steep hill toward the wooden Stone House where you will cross US 29 at the traffic light. This house, once a tavern, was transformed into an aide station during both battles. Cross a bridge and then continue walking up the hill. It's easy to imagine the battle in this large open field, a space with no place to hide.

Your last landmark is the Henry House, where disabled widow Judith Carter Henry lived with her daughter Ellen and a teenage slave named Lucy Griffith. Federal soldiers shot a cannon through the house, mortally wounding Judith. She was the battle's only known civilian casualty. Finish your hike at the visitor center.

NEARBY ACTIVITIES

Bull Run Winery is just a short drive from Manassas Battlefield. Time your visit around a show or concert at Jiffy Lube Live outdoor amphitheater. SplashDown Waterpark is a few miles away. Spend some time exploring charming downtown Manassas, a historic town with dozens of shops and restaurants. For another Civil War experience, visit Bristoe Station Battlefield Heritage Park in Bristow, Virginia.

• •

GPS TRAILHEAD COORDINATES N38° 48.773' W77° 31.287'

> **DIRECTIONS** From the Capital Beltway (I-495), take I-66 heading west. Drive 18 miles; then take Exit 47B toward VA 234 North. Merge onto VA 234 North; drive 1.7 miles to the Henry Hill Visitor Center at 6511 Sudley Road.

This hike takes you through fields, woods, wetlands, and multiple historic sites.

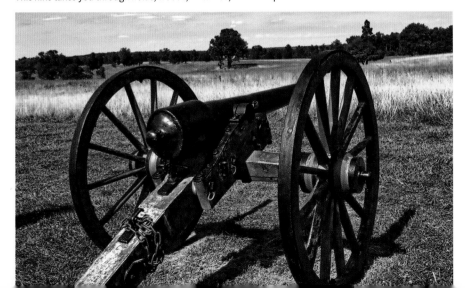

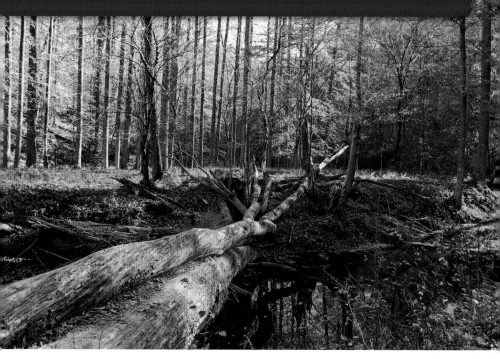

Enjoy the scenery as you walk along Quantico Creek through the park.

THIS HUGE NATURE PRESERVE provides a wonderful habitat for plants and wildlife. With 37 miles of hiking trails, there are easy and challenging routes to appeal to a wide range of hikers. This 6.2-mile hike offers a nice mix of terrain, including some wide-open roads as well as narrow pathways that overlook stream valleys. The most scenic section is along the Quantico Creek (along the South Valley and North Valley Trails). To shorten the hike, make it an out-and-back excursion along these two trails.

DESCRIPTION

Located about 20 miles southwest of the Capital Beltway, Prince William Forest Park ranks as the metro area's largest park. Covering 18,571 acres, it's also the largest woodland expanse within 50 miles of Washington. The area was well forested in pre-Colonial times, but more than two centuries of farming left the land badly eroded. In 1933 the federal government made it one of the country's 50 or so demonstration projects for restoring the environment and developing inexpensive recreation facilities. The Civilian Conservation Corps seeded slopes, created trails, and built facilities.

LENGTH 6.2 miles (with shorter options)

CONFIGURATION Loop

DIFFICULTY Moderate

SCENERY Rolling woodlands, stream valleys, waterfalls

EXPOSURE Partially open; more so in winter

TRAFFIC Usually light–very light; heavier in warm-weather season, especially on weekends and holidays

TRAIL SURFACE Dirt, with some rocky, rooty stretches; gravel and pavement

HIKING TIME 3.5 hours

DRIVING DISTANCE 33 miles

ACCESS Open daily, sunrise–sunset; entrance fee of $7 per vehicle

WHEELCHAIR TRAVERSABLE No

MAPS National Park Service, tinyurl.com /princewilliammap; also available at visitor center

FACILITIES Restrooms, water at trailhead

CONTACT National Park Service, 703-221-7181, nps.gov/prwi

LOCATION Triangle, Virginia

COMMENTS The trails are blazed and signposted but can be confusing to follow. Look for the concrete markers, and read the directional signs carefully. Be sure to stop at the visitor center to get a map before heading out. Make sure you have enough time to return before dark.

Eventually, in 1948, the area became a national park. Decades of recovery have transformed the depleted farmland. Trees, bushes, wildflowers, and ferns flourish, making springtime treks along the stream valleys a particular delight. Deer, beavers, squirrels, and other wildlife are plentiful. Their habitat extends into the adjoining Quantico Marine Corps Base, much of which is managed as a natural preserve.

To get started, park at the Pine Grove Picnic Area parking lot, located just west of the visitor center. The Laurel Trail Loop trailhead is located on the right side, beyond the picnic area. Enter the yellow- and blue-blazed dirt trail. At the first intersection, keep straight and cross the suspension footbridge. Turn left and walk along the wide gravel North Orenda Road until it ends. Turn right onto Scenic Drive (the park's major roadway). Walk in front of parking lot D, and then cross into the hiker-biker trail to proceed along the paved road to parking lot E. Turn right and walk through the parking lot to the trailhead, and then turn right into the woods and onto the Quantico Cascades Trail.

Then take a left at the next intersection onto Lake One Fire Road. The signage at the next intersection is a bit confusing; it says Geology Trail, which is not on the park's map. Take a left as the trail splits, and stay on the Quantico Cascades Trail until it becomes the Quantico Falls Trail and leads to the river. This yellow-blazed trail is a very narrow path through the woods and can be hard to see in fall when it is covered in leaves. This part of the park is heavily populated with mountain laurel, various oak species, and birch trees. It is also the steepest part of the hike, so watch your footing.

As you reach the river, turn left to view the Quantico Creek waterfalls. Then retrace your steps back to the right, and continue following the blue-blazed North

Prince William Forest Park

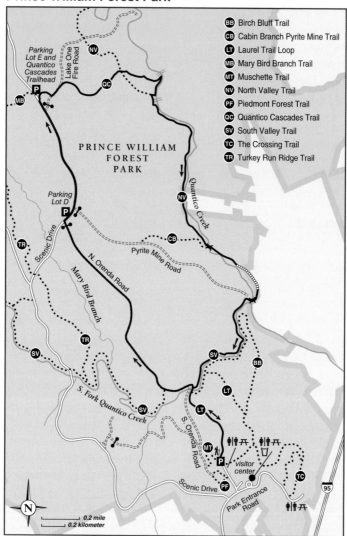

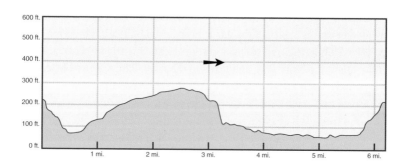

Valley Trail along the river, passing several small waterfalls along the way. Turn left to stay on the North Valley Trail, passing an overlook. The trail follows the river and then ascends high above the creek as you climb the valley wall. As you continue along the trail, you will pass the remains of the Cabin Branch Pyrite Mine. From 1889 to 1920, more than 200,000 long tons of pyrite were brought to the surface and processed into sulfuric acid to make soap, fertilizer, and gunpowder. The mine consisted of 70 buildings and employed 250 people. Today you can see some remains, although most of the land is now covered with Virginia pines.

Continue along the trail and at the bridge, turn left to cross over the creek toward the overlook and Pyrite Mine Road. Continue south on the other side of the stream, cross the boardwalk, and stop to enjoy the view from the overlook. Immediately after crossing a small bridge, take a sharp left onto the South Valley Trail. At the next intersection, turn right and then left across the suspension bridge on the Laurel Loop Trail. Retrace your steps straight ahead another 0.5 mile back to the Pine Grove parking lot.

NEARBY/RELATED ACTIVITIES

The park also offers bicycling, fishing, camping, and ranger-guided programs. Visit the nearby National Museum of the Marine Corps in Triangle, and explore the interactive exhibits that tell the story of the United States Marine Corps. Or head to historic Dumfries to visit the Weems-Botts Museum, where you will learn about the history of Virginia's oldest chartered town.

• •

GPS TRAILHEAD COORDINATES N38° 33.675' W77° 21.004'

DIRECTIONS From the Capital Beltway (I-495), take Exit 57A onto I-95 heading southwest toward Richmond. Take Exit 150B to VA 619. Head west on VA 619 (Joplin Road) 0.4 mile. Turn right onto the park entrance road.

Many small waterfalls flow across Quantico Creek through Prince William Forest Park.

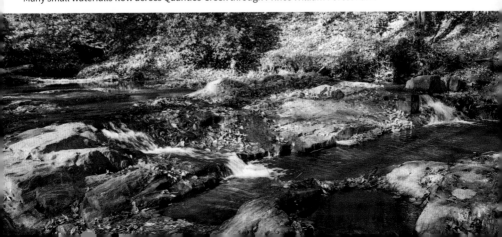

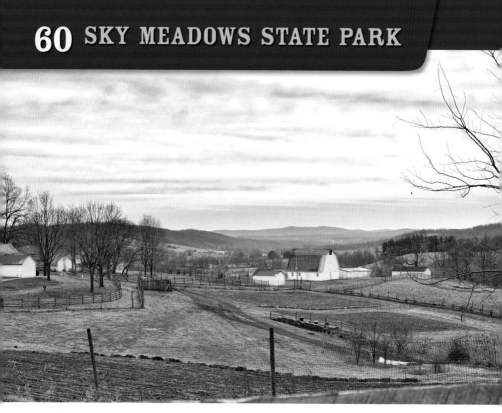

Surrounded by vineyards, Sky Meadows State Park is just 20 miles from the Front Royal entrance to Shenandoah National Park.

THIS STATE PARK in Virginia's portion of the Blue Ridge Mountains lives up to its name. Hikers can enjoy waterfalls, woodlands, vistas, exercise, and a visit to Virginia's wine country.

DESCRIPTION

Sky Meadows State Park, some 60 miles west of Washington, is located in Crooked Run Valley and is one of the farthest away of all our hikes. Suspended from the Appalachian Trail (AT), Sky Meadows spreads across the Blue Ridge's eastern flanks down to the Piedmont. It consists of almost nothing but slopes. The broad meadows are reminiscent of the Alps, with vistas unsurpassed in the metro area. The park has a wide array of trails with varying levels of difficulty, but most will cause you to break a sweat.

The 1,842-acre park lies within an extraordinary area of unspoiled and protected countryside along the border between Fauquier and Loudoun Counties. The landscape is one of woodlands and fields dotted with an occasional pond or farm building and crossed by a few ribbons of country road. It seems ageless, tranquil, and inviting. As farmland, the park's core area has a heritage dating back three centuries. A series of families raised crops, livestock, and children here. Their cumulative

LENGTH 3.6 miles (with longer options)

CONFIGURATION Loop

DIFFICULTY Moderate

SCENERY Vista-rich upland meadows; woodlands, waterfalls, farms, cattle, vineyards

EXPOSURE Some shade; some sun in open areas

TRAFFIC Light on weekdays; heavier on warm-weather weekends and holidays

TRAIL SURFACE Mostly dirt; some gravel and grass; rocky, rooty in places

HIKING TIME 2 hours (including time to view the overlook)

DRIVING DISTANCE 60 miles

SEASON Year-round

ACCESS Open daily, 8 a.m.–sunset; entrance fee

WHEELCHAIR TRAVERSABLE No

MAPS USGS *Upperville* and *Ashby Gap*; Potomac Appalachian Trail Club (PATC) Map 8; sketch map in free park pamphlet

FACILITIES Restrooms, water, phone at trailhead; gift shop

CONTACT Virginia Department of Conservation & Recreation, 540-592-3556, dcr.virginia.gov/state-parks/sky-meadows

LOCATION Delaplane, Virginia

COMMENTS This scenic park offers challenging climbs and may not be suitable for small children. Bring enough water and snacks, as concessions are limited.

history is preserved in the restored main building—called Mount Bleak—and other structures near the parking lot. Sky Meadows' beginnings as a park date back to the mid-1960s, when philanthropist and local resident Paul Mellon (son of Andrew, who gave us the National Gallery of Art and other treasures) saved the area from becoming an upscale subdivision. He donated the property to the State of Virginia in 1975. After the park was opened in 1983, the state added additional acreage to protectively encase a stretch of the AT. Later, the park grew to its present size when Mellon donated a 462-acre area just across US 17 for the use of horses and their riders.

Today, Sky Meadows is a beloved destination for hikers, picnickers, and photographers alike. It hosts regular events, including the Veterans Day 5K Run/Walk for Wounded Warriors, as well as nature and history programs. The park celebrates New Year's Day with a First Day Hike and offers family activities such as geocaching and Junior Ranger training.

The park has 24 miles of hiking trails and access to the AT. We chose this hike, a 3.6-mile loop that accumulates about 856 feet of elevation change, because it's a little easier for kids. The trail ascends above a farm that existed from Colonial to post–Civil War times until it reaches the North Ridge. You won't make it to the AT, but there are plenty of breathtaking views along the way. All the trails in Sky Meadows are named, color coded, well marked, well maintained, and well mapped. Be sure to stay on them when in the woods, where poison ivy lurks. In the meadows, steer clear of long grass to avoid ticks.

To get started from the parking-lot trailhead, head for the nearby park office building. Follow the dirt path about 140 yards, and then turn left onto Boston Mill

Sky Meadows State Park

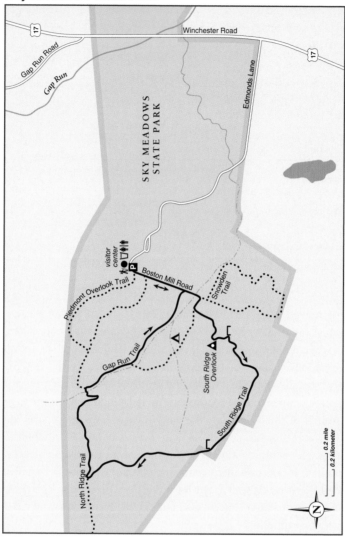

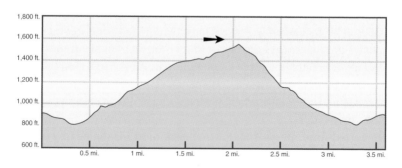

Road, a country lane where you'll rarely see a vehicle. Follow the lane gently downhill, past the Piedmont Overlook and Gap Run trailheads, and enter the yellow-blazed South Ridge Trail. There's a steady incline on this uneven, rocky trail, with lots of scrubby brush on either side. You'll see a streambed to your left and some old oak trees in the meadows. Follow the yellow blazes until you reach the South Ridge Overlook. Take a seat on the bench for a minute to enjoy the stunning view—barns, farmland, forests, and, in the distance, the Shenandoah Mountains.

Stay on the South Ridge Trail about 1.5 miles, detouring en route to catch your breath now and then. There's a second bench near the halfway point with another panoramic view and the Snowden Ruins (mounds of stones and what looks like it was once a fireplace). After the trail levels out somewhat and slides into the woods, you'll reach its T junction with the blue-blazed North Ridge Trail. Turn right and continue on the narrow, rocky trail as it heads gently back down the hill for nearly a mile (if you go left here, you'll meet up with the AT).

Following the blue blazes, you'll reach an intersection at the Gap Run Trail. Turn right and follow the orange blazes as this trail continues down the hill. There are a few fallen logs to cross over, giant boulders on the side of the trail, and uneven terrain that twists and turns. Soon you'll cross a stone bridge, placing the trail to the left of the stream that eventually turns into a waterfall. A metal fence protects hikers from the temptation to run into the tall grasses of the meadow.

As you near the end of Gap Run, you will see a little pond to your right. When you come to the Boston Mill Road, turn left to return the way you came, past the park office, and then turn right toward the parking lot.

Depending on the season and weather, you'll have views across the Piedmont to the east and south. Shorter hikes at Sky Meadows are worthwhile only if they include an overlook. For a vista-rich, 1-mile outing, just go up and down the Piedmont Overlook Trail.

NEARBY/RELATED ACTIVITIES

During the warm-weather months, tour Mount Bleak and sample the park's events and programs. Among them is the two-day Delaplane Strawberry Festival in late May; contact the park for details. Directly adjacent to the park are some vineyards worth a visit—Delaplane Cellars, Naked Mountain Winery, Three Fox, and RdV Vineyards. Close by, you'll find additional hiking opportunities at the Thompson Wildlife Management Area. From June to October, check out the family-run, pick-your-own orchards offering cherries, berries, and pumpkins (for details, visit pickyourown.org/vanorthern.htm). In July and August, the region's farms specialize in peaches, and in the fall, find more than 20 varieties of apple (plus fresh cider) at the Hartland-Troy Orchard, hartlandorchard.com.

• •

GPS TRAILHEAD COORDINATES N38° 59.572' W77° 58.046'

DIRECTIONS From the Capital Beltway (I-495) in Merrifield, Virginia, take Exit 49 to get on I-66 heading west. Proceed about 40 miles, and take Exit 23 onto US 17 north. Proceed 7.3 miles, and turn left into the park on Edmonds Lane. Drive 0.7 mile to the contact station and then 0.6 mile to the parking lot at the visitor center.

Located in Virginia's Piedmont region, in the foothills of the Blue Ridge Mountains, Sky Meadows is a beautiful place to spend the day hiking.

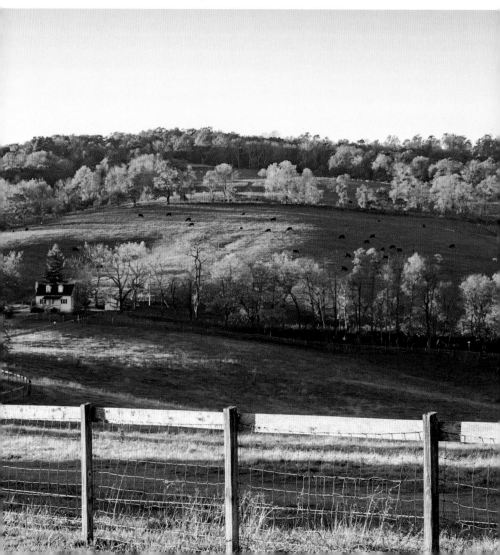

APPENDIX A: Hiking Clubs and Other Information Sources

All of the following regional or local organizations offer group day hikes year-round. Some of them also organize backpacking trips, bike rides, canoe outings, trail maintenance and other kinds of service trips, and social events. All of them post outing schedules on their websites.

APPALACHIAN MOUNTAIN CLUB, POTOMAC CHAPTER
outdoors.org/chapters/potomac

C & O CANAL ASSOCIATION
candocanal.org

CAPITAL HIKING CLUB
capitalhikingclub.org

CENTER HIKING CLUB
centerhikingclub.org

DC METROPOLITAN HIKERS
meetup.com/hiking-162

MARYLAND OUTDOOR CLUB
facebook.com/mdoutdoor

MID-ATLANTIC HIKING GROUP
meetup.com/mid-atlantic -hiking-group

MOSAIC OUTDOOR MOUNTAIN CLUB OF MARYLAND
mosaicmd.org

MOUNTAIN CLUB OF MARYLAND
mcomd.org

NORTHERN VIRGINIA HIKING CLUB
nvhc.com

NOVA TRAIL DOGS
meetup.com/activedogs-237

POTOMAC APPALACHIAN TRAIL CLUB
patc.net

SIERRA CLUB
   Washington, D.C., Chapter: dc.sierraclub.org

   Maryland Chapter: sierraclub.org /maryland

   Virginia Chapter: sierraclub.org /virginia

   Sierra Club Potomac Region Outings: sierraclub.org/virginia /potomac-region-outings

WANDERBIRDS HIKING CLUB
wanderbirds.org

WASHINGTON WOMEN OUTDOORS
washingtonwomenoutdoors.org

APPENDIX B: Hiking Stores

COLUMBIA SPORTSWEAR OUTLET
columbia.com

Tanger Outlets National Harbor
6800 Oxon Hill Road
Oxon Hill, MD 20745
301-965-9201

Clarksburg Premium Outlets
22705 Clarksburg Road, Ste. 630
Clarksburg, MD 20871

Leesburg Corner Premium Outlets
241 Fort Evans Road NE
Leesburg, VA 20176
571-293-3086

DICK'S SPORTING GOODS
dickssportinggoods.com

2470 Market St. NE
Washington, DC 20018
202-971-8214

5716 Columbia Pike
Bailey's Crossroads, VA 22041
703-933-0736

11160 Veirs Mill Road
Wheaton, MD 20902
301-933-3494

6601 Springfield Mall
Springfield, VA 22150
571-255-6367

2 Grand Corner Ave.
Gaithersburg, MD 20878
301-947-0200

EASTERN MOUNTAIN SPORTS
ems.com

200 Harker Place
Annapolis, MD 21401
410-573-1240

L.L. BEAN
llbean.com

8095 Tysons Corner Center
McLean, VA 22182
888-552-9876

MOUNTAIN TRAILS
mountain-trails.com

115 N. Loudoun St.
Winchester, VA 22601
540-667-0030

ORVIS
orvis.com

7000 Wisconsin Ave.
Bethesda, MD 20815
301-652-3562

THE NORTH FACE
thenorthface.com

3333 M St. NW
Washington, DC 20007
202-298-5510

OUTDOOR WORLD SPORTING GOODS
theoutdoorworld.com

Arundel Mills
7000 Arundel Mills Circle
Hanover, MD 21076
410-689-2500

PATAGONIA

patagonia.com

1048 Wisconsin Ave. NW
Washington, DC 20007
202-333-1776

REI CO-OP

rei.com

201 M St. NE
Washington, DC 20002
202-543-2040

910 Rose Ave.
North Bethesda, MD 20852
301-770-1751

8209 Watson St.
McLean, VA 22102
703-506-1938

3509 Carlin Springs Road
Bailey's Crossroads, VA 22041
703-379-9400

11950 Grand Commons Ave.
Fairfax, VA 22030
571-522-6568

15200 Potomac Town Place
Woodbridge, VA 22191
703-583-1938

INDEX